"It is not the strongest of the species that survives, nor the most intelligent. It is the one that is most adaptable to change." - Charles Darwin (attributed)

"You try to plant something in the concrete, y'know what I mean? If it grow, and the rose petal got all kind of scratches and marks, you not gonna say, 'Damn, look at all the scratches and marks on the rose that grew from concrete'; you gonna be like, 'Damn! A rose grew from the concrete?!'" – Tupac Shakur

The

Kitchen Sink Farming

Series

Volume 2: Fermenting [Edition 1]

Publisher:

Stone Soup Publications

Portland, OR 97239

publisher@KitchenSinkFarming.org

In humble gratitude to the trees that grew to make the paper recycled to make this book. I've tried to use you wisely.

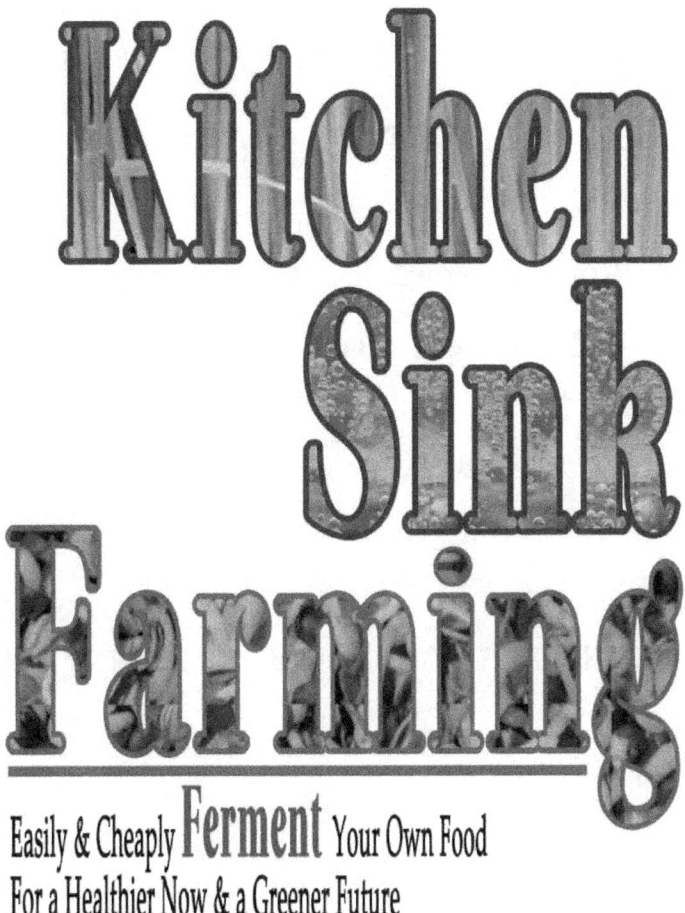

Kitchen Sink Farming

Easily & Cheaply **Ferment** Your Own Food
For a Healthier Now & a Greener Future

Volume 2

in the Kitchen Sink Farming Series

Jean-Pierre Parent

Also by Jean-Pierre Parent:

In the "Kitchen Sink Farming" Series:

- Vol 1: Sprouting

- Vol 2: Fermenting

- Vol 3: Growing

- Vol 4: Homegrown Living Recipes - What to Do with Your Sprouts and Krauts

- The Complete Set: all 4 Volumes

and

Practice Makes… Meditation and Yoga in Everyday Life

JP's blogs

Food: www.KitchenSinkFarming.org

Yoga: www.OmInvasion.org

Contents

Preface

This book is the result of a serious personality flaw.

Somehow, from a very early age, I've rarely been satisfied with anything. Or, more accurately, I'm only satisfied with perfection, that acutely rare and delicate moment when the stars align; the air is just so, filling the lungs with sweet fortitude and the project before you sparkles with temporal rightness…

This eternal dissatisfaction with the lack of perfection pervades every aspect of my life: my athleticism, health, relationships, even conversations. I practice them beforehand, and I think about them afterwards, re-working them in my mind until my responses are the most thoughtful, compassionate, wise, and considerate statements possible.

As a little kid playing with my Atari, I hit the reset button on the console more often than the one on the controller, restarting the game over and over if I did something that wasn't *quite* right, so that I could have another chance to do it again, only this time, perfectly. At the time, I think I expected all of life could be like that.

But I think I really hit my "always-satisfied-with-the-best" stride with food. If I was eating something (and that happened quite often in those days), I would wonder "what's the best possible form of this food?" So I cut out junk food and soda (I think I was nine at this time), after experiencing how I felt after eating a fast food hamburger before a soccer game. Didn't make that mistake again. I soon came to learn about vegetarian, then vegan, then organic, then raw food. The quest didn't stop there though, because of the widely varying ideas of raw vs. living food, organic standards, and genetic modification of food. Recently, the world's largest chain of natural food grocery stores was caught selling frozen vegetables as organic that were actually grown in China with little respect for chemical-free farming, and the "independent" organic certifiers that permitted the labeling are owned by the store (more on pg 27). So it's a constant question about who's trustworthy, and "how long will they be?" (See chapter "Truly Empty Calories", subchapter "When Organic Isn't (It's Too Easy Being Green)" for more on this particular paranoia).

Then there is the immeasurable question of taste. All this wholesome and nutritious food (much like the bland and boring natural choices offered when I was a kid, and 90% of them today) might be good for the body but unless it can create sublime waves of closed-eye, headed-tilted moaning pleasure, it does little for the soul. And therefore leaves something to be desired. Incomplete. Imperfect.

These days, my slightly mellowed aspirations for perfection have made me an experimenter, a scientist, a chef, a do-it-yourself-er. Before sitting down to write this (at a desk that I built so I could be the perfect height, with a pillow that I cut from the perfect density of memory foam mattress, on which I am sitting in a yoga position called siddhasana, or perfect pose), I noticed that some pumpkin seeds I sprouted and put in my dehydrator for a crunchy snack were sticking together. Makes sense, if you've ever lobotomized a pumpkin for a jack-o-lantern, scooping out its slimy stuck-together seeds. I thought that

> "I have simple tastes. I am always satisfied with the best."
> – Oscar Wilde

natural cohesion might be a good start to a flatbread, maybe mixed with super-sticky flax. So, did I make *a* pumpkinseed-flax flatbread? No… I made about 2 dozen. Equal parts flax and pumpkin. Double one, and double the other. Each one of those split in thirds, one part put on the counter to ferment, one in the oven at a low temp, and the rest in the dehydrator at a lower temp. Each of *those* split in half again, dry or with some oil. One in each category blended with some sprouted spelt, to see if they'd be better a little cake-ier. All labeled and catalogued. You get the idea.

Some may think that this level of precision is boring, rigid, anal-retentive, or obsessive, and I might agree if it was focused on a less important subject. But I think nourishment is just too important to be satisfied with anything less than utterly thorough knowledge, which until recently we've had to mostly figure out by our lonesomes. I think that this mindset is an integral part of being able to draw the measure of life's awesomeness and maybe the best way to experience the most happiness, fun, health, contentedness, and eventual freedom, because I will *know* what the best choice is for me today. With certainty. That's the goal, anyways. And then I'm happy, because the mundane turns into magic when it's dove into with attentive and receptive enthusiasm.

This book is the result of my decades-long experiment that asks the question: what's the best food possible, to fuel the best life possible? I think I've found glimmers of the answer, and I'm so pleased to be able to share them with you.

This is what led me to eating whole, organic, living foods: wanting to get as much out of my food as possible. Your reasons might be totally different. Starting with pure ingredients is a life-saver for someone with food allergies – the only way to take control of what goes into your body. Even someone lactose intolerant can enjoy the bowel-healing properties of milk (as raw kefir), butter (as ghee), or cheeses of many kinds (all in Kitchen Sink Farming Volume 2: Fermenting). Cancer patients find remission through fermented foods. The environmental benefits of enough home growers and sprouters will have a major global impact. A network of neighbors, each specializing in a different product could build a community like nothing else – focusing around the most primal and fundamental cement of society. And as I'll mention time and again, it's also the cheapest way to eat what is possibly the very best food in the world.

The "Why?"

The world's best foods aren't available in stores. You can't get them from the home shopping network, either. It's a good thing, too, because then people would buy them and miss out on the particular satisfaction of eating something they grew themselves, acutely aware of the life cycle of and organic rhythms of nature in their current mouthful. It's also a good thing because they're really cheap and really easy to make. Once you try it, it'd be laughable to pay someone else to do it. This book is based on the firm fact that anyone, anywhere, at any time, can be enjoying a bounty of fresh, living, incredibly nutritious food with very little work and expense.

Once you've enjoyed a delicious and vibrant lunch made from sprouted seeds, grains, or nuts bursting with taste and life, you won't need any convincing. You'll know by that point how easy, cheap, and fun it is to grow sweet strawberries, succulent micro greens, and juicy tomatoes with shocking depth of flavor in your seventh-story apartment kitchen, washing them down with home-brewed, wild-yeasted ginger ale or sparkling kombucha tea. In the meantime, though, before you figure all

> "A great revolution in just one single individual will help achieve a *change* in the destiny of a society and, further, will enable a *change* in in the destiny of humankind."
> *Daisaku Ikeda*

that out for yourself, it's supportive to know exactly why you're doing what you're doing. Maybe you're interested in increasing the amount of fresh, organic food you're eating (and there's no fresher food than something grown 5 feet away from your table and "picked" when you take your first chew!) and dramatically improving your health, energy, and immune system. Maybe you want to save money on groceries or have less of an impact on the earth, casting a vote against industrialized, destructive modern farming methods. Or maybe girls (and guys) just wanna have fun in the kitchen. Whatever your reason, learning about the myriad benefits of sprouting, indoor gardening, and fermenting at home will only encourage and inspire. And it just might make you able to explain to your mom why the dinner peas have leaves.

Nutrients and enzymes don't take kindly to cooking, canning, or sitting on shelves. Even fresh, organic produce loses valuable benefits every hour it's wilting away under the grocery store lights. In Los Angeles, it's hard to walk a few blocks and not pass a Whole Foods or organic restaurant. But even there, in the city with perhaps the greatest access to all things health, sprouted peanut butter, Kamut grass juice (wheat's superior ancestor), unpasteurized sauerkraut, enzymatically-active hot soups, and raw goat milk kefir are either not for sale, or else have to be painstakingly and expensively tracked down, even though they require very little knowledge, no expensive equipment, and less than a minute a day to make. When I was learning the things in this book, even though my efforts usually required a lot of trial and error, I kept coming back to the same eureka feeling: "It *can't* be this easy." But it is. A short and hopefully fun learning adventure will have you eating better than ever before, saving money, and feeling amazing. Maybe one day your local Piggly Wiggly will have a nut butter cafe, where they'll grind the freshly sprouted nuts of your choice, which you can spread on the apple a polite and well-groomed apron-clad deli worker just picked in front of you. If, and when we get there, through the slow and painstaking process of transforming consumer opinion and convincing the huge conglomerates that it's cost-effective to service us in this way, they'll surely charge an arm and a snout for it. No. The only way to eat living, vital, delicious food is to grow and prepare it yourself.

Nerd Corner!

Sprouting seeds increases their nutrient availability by 50-2000%, with an average of about 500%. See table on pages 14-15 to see the effects on specific nutrients after sprouting mung beans (not the most common spout, but possibly the most fun to say).

Nature is a hard-working and dedicated employee. Hire her to work for you and then sit back and relax. Nobody fertilizes or irrigates the forest. It's a complete system that does these things on its own. Make a "food forest" in your apartment, home, or patio, and your main effort is to pick the food. You put in some effort at the very beginning, but once the system is established, you work a lot less. You could call Kitchen Sink Farming "lazy agriculture", because you're working *with* nature, and not against her. You're using the laws of nature, forces that apply equally on a rainforest floor, a Brooklyn backyard, or a Tokyo high-rise to grow your lunch. Sprouting, fermenting, and growing your own food are plain and simply the best foods you can get. They require the least amount of energy to digest, contain the most nutrition, and have the least impact on the environment, resources, and humanity, providing for the longest, most disease and discomfort-free life. And wouldn't you know it: it's the cheapest and easiest way to create food, too. Anyone in the world can apply at least one principal in this book, and the more you work into your own everyday life, the better off that life will be for it.

Sprouting: Why Mess with a Perfectly Good Seed?

1) Sprouting activates enzymes.

Sprouts have an average of 7 times the number of enzymes needed to digest them, enzymes that can go to work digesting other foods, repairing and regenerating the body. See "Kitchen Sink Farming Vol 4: Homegrown Living Recipes - What to Do with Your Sprouts and Krauts" for more on enzymes.

"Intelligence is the ability to adapt to change."
Stephen Hawking

2) Sprouting Increases Nutrition.

Sprouted seeds supply nutrients in a predigested form – food is broken down into its simplest and easiest-to-digest components. During sprouting, much of the starch is broken down into simple sugars such as glucose and sucrose by the action of the enzyme 'amylase'. Proteins are converted into amino acids and amides. Fats and oils are converted into more simple fatty acids by the enzyme lipase. Sprouts are also high in fiber, so that along with their water content are even more helpful with digestion.

3) Sprouting Removes "Enzyme Inhibitors".

Enzyme Inhibitors keep seeds from sprouting at the wrong time, and keep nutrients locked up. Sprouting seeds also makes them easier to digest and more nutritious for this reason, actually making everything you eat before and after more nutritious too. (see pg 67 for more)

Table 1: Effects of Sprouting on Mung Beans

First two columns of chart reprinted from <u>Critical Reviews in Food Science and Nutrition,</u> 1989; 28(5):401-37. "Nutritional improvement of cereals by sprouting", <u>Chavan JK</u>, <u>Kadam SS</u>., Department of Biochemistry, Mahatma Phule Agricultural University, Rahuri, India.

Protein	Increases 30%	The increase in protein availability is an indicator of the overall enhancement of nutritional value of a sprouted seed.
Carbohydrates	Decreases 15%	The simultaneous reduction in carbohydrate and caloric content indicates that many carbohydrate molecules are broken down during sprouting to allow absorption of atmospheric nitrogen to reform it into amino acids. The resulting protein is the most easily digestible of all proteins.
Calcium	Increases 30%	
Potassium	Increases 80%	
Sodium	Increases 690%	The skyrocketing sodium content is a good indication that foods are much

		more easily digestible in the sprouted form, as sodium is essential to the digestive process, particularly in the intestines, and also to the elimination of carbon dioxide. The building blocks of both nutrition and digestibility peak simultaneously.
Iron	Increases 40%	
Vitamin A	Increases 285%	
Vitamin B1 (Thiamine)	Increases 208%	
Vitamin B2 (Riboflavin)	Increases 515%	
Vitamin B3 (Niacin)	Increases 256%	
Vitamin C	Infinite Increase	Dry seeds don't show a measurable amount of Vitamin C, but it skyrockets when they're sprouted. Vitamin C is important in the metabolization of proteins, which also increase in sprouted seeds.

A Deeper Reason to Take Control of Our Food: Truly Empty Calories

Food that's not organically grown by traditional, natural methods (paradoxically called "conventionally-grown") is fairly devoid of nutrients. Large-scale commercial farmers discovered in the 1940's that three nutrients are required to grow and produce normal-looking crops: nitrogen, phosphorous, and potassium, or NPK, but plants, like us, require over 100 minerals to be at their best, and if it's not in the soil, it's not on your plate. Plants grown "conventionally" don't have the nutrients they need to develop healthy immune systems, requiring farmers to spray them down with a heavy coat of pesticides, herbicides, and fungicides. When we eat the fruit and vegetables that come off of nutrient-deficient, chemical pesticide-laden plants, we suffer in two ways: very little nutrition and a dose of cancer-causing chemicals. When I'm travelling and can't get organic produce, I feel as if I'm eating photographs of food. The apples look like apples, they're red and round, but they're tasteless and my body feels a lifeless chunk of food in my belly as if I've been chewing on paper. My body is waiting for the flood of nourished happiness that it's used to, but doesn't come.

It gets worse. Turns out this disconnect is the well-planned stratagem of big business, that can almost always be counted on to put profits before people. Consumers are starting to become aware of a decades-old curtain of misinformation and propaganda drawn between grocery store shoppers and the contents of their carts by

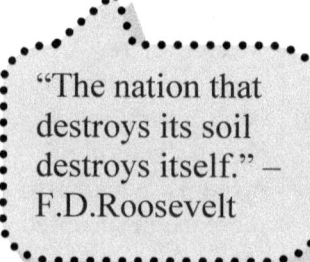

"The nation that destroys its soil destroys itself." – F.D.Roosevelt

massive agribusiness and its bigger, cheaper, faster business model. But it wasn't always this way.

A History of Agri-Tech

Before World War II, people farmed the way they always have: fertilizing their fields with nutrient-dense organic matter or growing where rivers overflow and deposit the year's worth of mineral-rich silt. They rotated crops so plants that take certain nutrients from the soil are supported by a season of plants that put those nutrients back. They relied on the strength of the crops' own immunity to fight off pests. Rainbows glittered over every dew-speckled family-farmed field of organic heirloom veggies… Ok, not really, but food *was* more nutritious and less carcinogenic.

> "Humanity consumed 120% of the earth's sustainable resource capacity in 1999" - National Academy of Sciences, June 2007

World War II inspired many advances in industrial science, from napalm and synthetic rubber to the atomic bomb. When it was over, huge stocks of nitrates from ammunition building, organophosphates for making nerve gas, and other chemicals had accumulated. Nitrates contain nitrogen, one component of the NPK triad, and an enterprising chemical company re-labeled them "fertilizer". Nerve agents like mustard gas, shown to block communication between the brain and organs in both humans and insects alike, were called "pesticides", and both of these were sold to post-war farms. These chemicals, with only slight variations are still used today, and over 1.5 million pounds of organophosphates are sprayed every year on California farms alone.

The huge demand placed on modern farmers to feed more and more people on less and less space is creating an unparalleled desperation. In an attempt to keep up with demand, farmers have fired nature and are courting the promise of a dangerous and only partially-understood technology.

Burger & a Side of Flies: Genetic Modification of Food

Pick a single-ingredient food off the supermarket shelves and you have a 70% chance of grabbing a genetically modified organism, or GMO. This is the volatile and very scary process of splicing a fruit, veggie, or grain's DNA with genes from another organism, always part bacteria, often animal and sometimes even insect, human, or virus. Choose something with corn (or a derivative like corn syrup, dextrose, baking powder, caramel and caramel coloring, mono and diglycerides, modified food starch, vegetable anything: broth, oil, protein, shortening, and the many other ways industrious food scientists have found to pump the most heavily-subsidized and therefore most commonly-grown crop in the US into our diets) or a food with more than a few ingredients and unless it's organic or specifically labeled "non-GMO", your chances of choosing a genetically modified organism go up to around 100%. The ancient process of plant breeding is this: put two plants with traits you like next to each other and hope they'll cross-pollinate and the next generation will be an even better plant.

This wasn't precise or fast enough for modern agri-business. GMO was born out of the desire to achieve total dominion over crops, under the guise of lowering costs and increasing yields. But as with the attempt to control most things in nature, the outcome was not the expected one. Genetic modification has actually cost agriculture more, after recalls on untamable seeds, the inability of GM plants to access nutrients in the soil, puzzlingly lower yields in drought conditions and increased needs for more powerful pesticides with the consequence of mutant super-weeds. None of these issues have impeded cell-invasive technology's expansion, however, as the planting of GM crops went from zero acres in 1988 to 3.7 million in 1996 to 100 million in 2003. Most of the financial burden has fallen not on the slick-talking companies, however, but on the farmers who were taken in by their glimmering promises. It becomes a deadly gamble when, like between 2001 and 2005, 32,000 Indian farmers committed suicide underneath the avalanche of debt an Indian subsidiary of the Monsanto Corporation pawned off onto them when their GM cotton fields were ravaged by a disease that affected only GM plants. Ironically, at least one of the farmers killed himself, at 25 years old, by drinking a liter of pesticide.

Monsanto is one of the companies that is single-handedly destroying the traditional methods of farming in favor of a near-fascist domination of farmers and the very DNA of the seeds they plant, and along with it the worlds' food supply. Monsanto, whose first success was Agent Orange, the forest defoliant used in the Vietnam War are and has since been found guilty in Federal courts of falsifying their earnings statements (Foreign Corrupt Practices Act (15 U.S.C. § 78dd-1)), bribing government officials around the globe (15 U.S.C § 78m(b)(2) & (5)), knowingly polluting the small town of Anniston, Alabama, with dangerous levels of polychlorinated biphenyls (PCBs) resulting in over 3.500 cases of cancer and other degenerative diseases, mislabeling pesticides to minimize their dangers (*Monsanto guilty of chemical poisoning in France,* Reuters Feb 13, 2012) and countless other crimes against humankind and nature. In the year 2000, it was estimated that 10 new people everyday are diagnosed with cancer due to exposure to dioxin produced by Monsanto (US Environmental Protection Agency's (EPA) draft reassessment on dioxin) and as of this writing, Monsanto is being taken to court by a group of Argentinean tobacco farmers who say that the biotech giant knowingly poisoned them with herbicides and pesticides and subsequently caused "devastating birth defects" in their children.

But the *really* scary part of this whole mess is that these "franken-foods" reproduce in unexpected and uncontrollable ways. Bizarre monstrosities of barely recognizable plants discovered in fields. 1000-generational heirloom corn farms contaminated by invading mutant DNA. Monsanto's BT corn, cotton, and soy are *themselves*

"A molecular study conducted by Mexican, American and Dutch researchers demonstrates the presence of genes from genetically modified organisms (GMO) among the varieties of traditional corn cultivated in the remote regions of Oaxaca State in the southern part of the country, even though the Mexican government has always maintained a moratorium on the use of transgenic seed." - from "GMO Contamination in Mexico's Cradle of Corn" *Le Monde*, December 11 2008

registered as pesticides. The process of genetically modifying foods is not only unethical and disgusting, but we're messing with forces we don't understand and the current results are hinting at world-wide epidemics of sci-fi horror film proportions. For example, in 1989 there was an outbreak of a new disease in the US, traced back to a batch of an L-tryptophan food supplement produced with GMO bacteria. Though it contained less than .1% of the highly toxic compound, 37 people died that year and 1,500 were left with permanent disabilities.

The Food and Drug Administration declared that it was not gene modification that was at fault but a failure in the purification process. However, the company concerned, Showa Denko, admitted that the low-level purification process had been used without ill effect in non-GM batches. Scientists at Showa Denko blame the GM process for producing traces of a potent new toxin, and this new toxin had never been found in non-GM versions of the product. In May 2008, new findings by the Physicians and Scientists for Responsible Application of Science and Technology (PSRAST) caused them to state, "Most importantly, the poison considered

"Typically, if something is to be considered Generally Recognized as Safe (G.R.A.S.) it needs lots of peer-reviewed published studies and an overwhelming consensus among the scientific community. With GM crops, they had neither."
– Jeffrey Smith, author, *Seeds of Deception*

most important in the tryptophan was closely similar to tryptophan (a dimer), but never found in natural bacteria. This indicates that disturbed tryptophan metabolism generated the poison. Moreover, the inserted genes were directed at altering the metabolism (so as to increase tryptophan production).

Our conclusion is that the only plausible explanation for the appearance of this poison is disturbances of the natural metabolic processes due to genetic engineering."

This is just one example of the dangers of genetic manipulation. It's easy to imagine that every instance of genetic modification has its own tale, or will. In fact, children have more adverse reactions to GMOs than adults, and it's hard to not picture a future without horrible consequences from freely fucking with nature.

From news footage of Vice President George Bush Sr. at the Monsanto factory in 1987:

Monsanto Executive: "We have no complaint about the way the USDA is handling it; they're going through an orderly process… Now if we're waiting til September and we don't have our authorization we may say something different!"

Bush: "Call me. We're in the de-reg [de-regulation] business. Maybe we can help."

The idea hits home even harder when a public official in Japan, where GM foods are outlawed stated their plan to "watch US children for the next ten years" before they determine their next course of action, according to the documentary "The Future of Food" (Deborah Koons Garcia, Lily Films, 2004).

Bio-engineered foods don't have, and were never designed, to provide any benefit to the consumer. No attempt has been made to make more nutritious wheat or better-tasting spinach. Instead, the GM industry's only goal is profit (of everyone but the farmer), so the scam has been sold to the American consumer as a way to provide food for the masses of overpopulated future generations. One problem with this logic is that the nearly 1 billion malnourished people (10,000 of which die every day from starvation) don't do so because of a lack of food. Many of these people used to be farmers, but were kicked off their land when their respective governments accepted huge loans from multi-national banks, and subsistence farming wasn't a workable way to pay them back. Forced off their farms and into the slums of industrializing third-world cities, they have gone from being food independent to food-dependant. The calamitous issue of world hunger is not a problem of production; it's a crisis of access, which is strange when one considers that the average piece of food travels 1500 miles from the farm to the supermarket. The other argument with this propaganda is Monsanto's plan to include in all seeds they produce a "terminator gene", a self-destructing abomination that creates a plant with sterile progeny. That means that if you buy a seed from Monsanto and plant it, instead of being able to harvest the seeds from your plants for next year, you will have to buy more seeds. This is clear proof that the biotech industry has no interest in "feeding the world", as their propaganda states. In the same way that GMO seeds have mysteriously found their way into native plant genes (see quote below), the danger of this terminator gene out-crossing into the plants that make up the world's food supply, effectively ending traditional, sustainable farming, must have gone unnoticed by the company's scientists and members of the USDA who both approved the use of the gene and co-own it. No one can be that evil.

But who is responsible if terminator genes cross-contaminate unsuspecting food supplies? By past precedent, it's not the seed company that's to blame but the farmer, and courts have told farmers that by not protecting their fields properly from seeds blowing in (an absolutely ludicrous idea), they have unwittingly signed a contract with the biotech company that's patented that specific invading gene. Is it possible that one day the world's entire food supply will be controlled by the company that brought us PCB's (which are present in the cells of every man, woman, and child on Earth), DDT, bovine growth hormone, and dioxins, and who has bribed government officials to look the other way while illegally dumping 50 tons of mercury into one Alabama river, stating "We cannot afford to lose one dollar of business", in an internal memo (a leaked copy of which is readily available online) found when this criminal polluting was exposed?

"AG Biotech will find a supporter occupying the White House next year, regardless of which candidate wins the election in November."
– Monsanto In-House Newsletter, Oct 6, 2000, in reference to the multiple White House officials that are also board members of Monsanto.

Monsanto does, however, have most of America's, and soon the world's, farmers completely dependent on them each planting season. And their wrath is swift and brutal against farmers even suspected of saving viable seeds. Even farmers with neighboring fields that have had these manipulated genes carried by the wind into their crops, which then cross into the genes of the new plants, are pressured with debilitating lawsuits to either go out-of-business or sign a contract and enter into the cycle of dependence and perversion.

Not surprisingly, by current FDA regulations, GMO foods aren't allowed to be labeled as such.

"We received over 44,000 pages from the FDA's own files and they revealed that the FDA has been lying to the world since 1992, if not before. But they continue to lie, they're still lying, they claim that there's an overwhelming consensus in the scientific community that genetically engineered foods are as safe as their conventionally produced counterparts and they claim that there has been sufficient data to back up this consensus. [Based on the FDA files] both of those claims are blatant lies." Steven Druker, lawyer for the Alliance for Bio-Integrity, who forced the FDA to unclassify its internal files on GMOs.

And back to the history... After WWII, famers began growing just one crop on a field, requiring more and more chemical support as the malnourished plants weakened. In fact, according to the National Resources Defense Council, pesticide use since the 1940's has gone up 10 times, but crop loss due to insects has doubled, and in the meantime, the Environmental Protection Agency estimates that there are pesticide residuals in the tissues of every American. Our current agricultural system now relies on toxic fertilizers to keep the land producing food, as the precious topsoil that took thousands of years to develop is being washed

"This [genetic modification of food] is the largest biological experiment humanity has ever entered into." – Dr. Ignacio Chapel, Microbial Biologist, UC Berkeley

away at an alarming rate. In fact, in the last 50 years, America has lost over 75% of its fertile soil. It takes 200 to 1000 years to create just one inch of topsoil; no modern technology can make it faster than that. Add to that the fact that the world's main food-producing countries like the US, China, India, Australia and Spain have or are about to reach their water resource limits, and you have an unsustainable agricultural system that can't go on this way much longer. Our dependence on chemical agriculture is a slippery slope. Like hard drugs, we need more and more to get the same effects. Something's gotta give, or soon there will be no seeds to sow, no topsoil to sow them in, no water to water them with, and certainly no way to protect them from the very gentlest of bugs. The only way out is for you and me to take responsibility for what we're putting into our bodies by growing it ourselves, not just voting for change but passionately and peacefully dissenting against an untenable system by planting or sprouting a seed and eating it with delight.

There is hope that the US will follow the example of Europe and Japan who, not beholden to the rebates, subsidies, and political and collegiate contributions of the biotech industries, have outlawed all GM foods. A federal judge recently invalidated the patent on a gene that is known to cause breast cancer, owned by Myriad Genetics in association with the University of Utah, who charged exorbitant fees to research facilities using the gene to research breast cancer prevention. This ruling casts doubt on the motives of the companies holding gene patents and raises important ethical questions about the ability to patent life.

When Organic Isn't (It's too easy being green)

Obviously, it's better to buy organic food over conventional. It's a vote for the health of your family, your community, and the environment.
Unfortunately, just choosing produce with an organic sticker isn't enough. I want to believe the strict and stringent guidelines for organic certification

"If we're still dragging our feet in 2015, it really becomes almost impossible for the world to avert a degree of climate change that we simply will not be able to manage", John Holdren, Professor of Environmental Policy, Harvard University, and Director of the White House Office of Science and Technology Policy

are followed by participating farms with enthusiasm and far-sighted wisdom, but I know too much about the funding the certifiers receive from the corporations whose goal it is to relax the laws for the betterment of their immediate profits. I hear too many stories from friends in the biz who are told to slap an organic sticker on every fifth crate of asparagus they're packing and call it a day. In 2005 in the UK, the widespread epidemic of fraudulently labeling meat as organic was a scandal that required a major government crackdown. The USDA, America's main certification agency who both makes the rules and sells organic certification, is heavily funded by Monsanto and other biotech conglomerates. It's companies like these that are fighting for (and paying for) more lenient rules within an increasingly lucrative market.

And it's working: a 2006 amendment created a list of 38 synthetic ingredients allowed in products that can still be called organic. This allowed Anheuser-Busch in 2007 to have its "Wild Hop Lager" certified organic even though it uses hops grown with chemical fertilizers and sprayed with pesticides. Advocacy groups fear that, since almost all organic foods are now sold through high-volume distribution channels like Target and Wal-Mart (the #1 retailer of organics in the US), the laws will change to support the massive producers, and the small farms that pioneered traditional methods of farming will be squeezed out. While they wait for the laws to change, Wal-Mart continually pressures their suppliers to cut corners, if not to break laws outright. In 2007, Aurora Organic Dairy, Wal-Mart's main supplier of organic dairy products, was found to be in violation of 14 organic regulations and would have lost their certification if it weren't for some unusual leniency on the part of the FDA. The truth is, the organic label can be bought, and is at best a vague indication of standards practiced in fields and facilities. On the other side of the coin, many small farms that operate according to organic guidelines and beyond aren't certified simply because they can't afford to be.

The simple truth is that big business cannot be trusted to do the right thing when millions or billions of dollars are at stake. Advertisers use buzz words like "fresh", "family-owned", "natural", or "local", not in an effort to accurately describe, but to sell with little interest in the truth. It's gotten quite out of hand how advertisers can say absolutely anything and we, in our nose-to-the-grindstone haste to feel better, or check "good for us" off of our grocery lists, let ourselves be unthinkingly swayed.

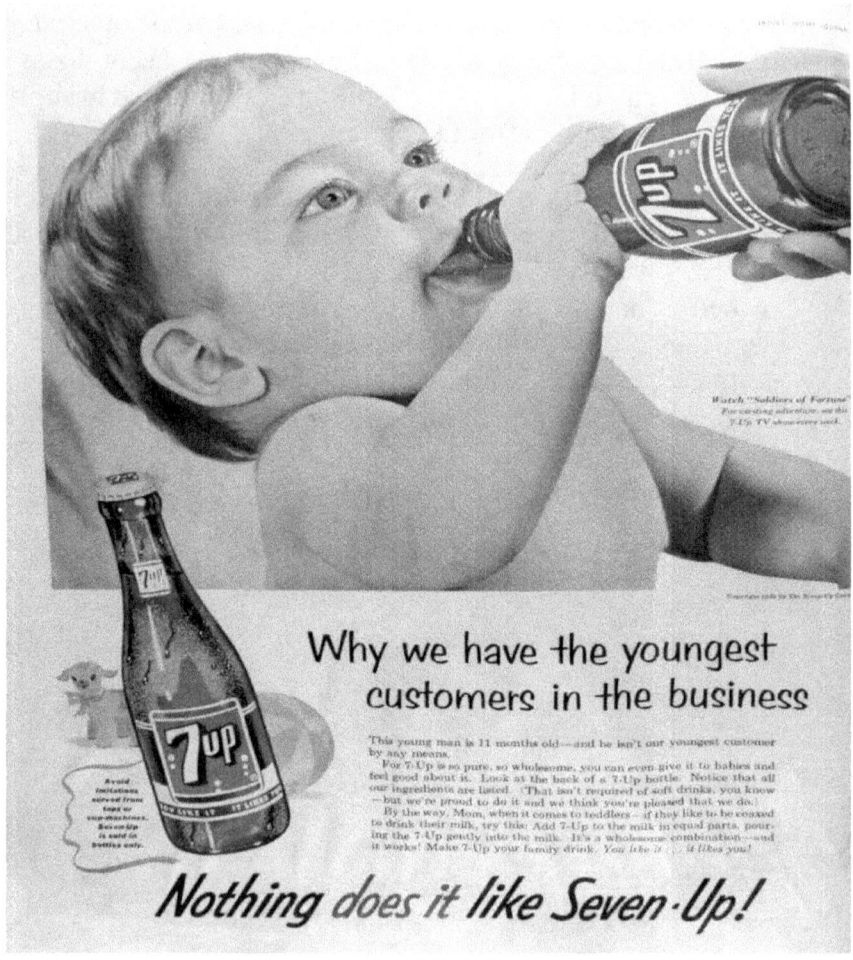

A would-be-funny-if-it-wasn't-so-sad example of deceptive 1955 advertising. Will we look back in 50 years with an equally ironic sophistication to Wendy's "You Know When It's Real" campaign, Nestle's "eco-shaped bottled water", and the other 98% of products world-wide tested in 2009 (by TerraChoice, who runs the Environmental Choice Program for the Canadian government) whose labels were found to be misleadingly green-washed?

Recently, the world's largest chain of natural food grocery stores came under fire for misrepresenting the quality of their store-brand frozen organic vegetables. Turns out the "Organic California Blend", as well as snap peas, spinach, and some others, were produced in China, and the store misleadingly and illegally put "USDA Organic" and "QAI" (Quality Assurance International) stamps on the foods, though neither organization had inspected the farms or food. They have, however, inspected hundreds of tons of food grown in China that were contaminated with chemicals and/or pathogens.

These stories shed light on the dark corners of the entire organic movement, which retailers like Whole Foods have ridden to massive financial success. Agriculture giants like Gerber's, Heinz, *Dole,* ConAgra and ADM, who have no problem poisoning workers, consumers, and the Earth with toxic chemical practices have jumped on the bandwagon with Earthy-friendly sounding organic subsidiaries. It takes little common sense to realize that massive conglomerates, who commonly purchase pesticides that have been outlawed in the US to use in their South American plants before shipping them back to American consumers (a bizarre loophole in the law), can't be trusted to make ethical decisions about my food when one simple lie can net them

"If people let government decide what foods they eat, their bodies will soon be in as sorry a state as are the souls of those who live under tyranny." –Thomas Jefferson

millions of dollars. Same goes for Target, recently sued for mislabeling natural products like rice milk and tofu as organic. Or that, though "organic farm" and "small family farm" are interchangeable in most consumers' minds, almost all the organic food produced in America comes from California, where 5 or 6 huge operations dominate the market. 80% of US beef is produced by 4 companies[1]. The vast majority of the seeds planted by the world's farmers come from 4 conglomerations of companies. Food retailers are also on a consolidation track. By some estimates, within the next ten years all of the retail food in the world will be controlled by 6 companies, only one of which will be American, Wal-Mart. Represent! This means that the selection and labeling of products on your grocery store shelves will be decided by a broker, potentially on another continent, based on what will return the largest profit.

If you sprout and grow your own food, you know it's organic. If you buy it, you only hope it is.

Home growing, sprouting, and fermenting is one of the best ways to take responsibility for your own health and impact on the environment, and creates a haven from the conspiracy of corporate greed and consumer manipulation that plays like a Hollywood movie. The few seconds it takes to rinse our sprouts can re-establish our primordial bond to the land, the elements, and the moment-to-moment birth, maturation, and transformation of the pulsating forces of life around us. Even 100 glass and steel stories above the cement, life presses powerfully on. All this from an unused

---

[1] Nebraska and S Dakota passed constitutional amendments banning all farms not family-owned. Corporate agri-business didn't like that one bit, but state constitutions (and government in general) are in fact of, by, and for the people. Oops.

square-foot spot on a kitchen counter or closet shelf that would otherwise be collecting dust or worse, historical spoons from ebay.

Collapse, the Future of Food

"A living planet is a much more complex metaphor for deity than just a bigger father with a bigger fist. If an omniscient, all-powerful Dad ignores your prayers, it's taken personally. Hear only silence long enough, and you start wondering about his power. His fairness. His very existence. But if a world mother doesn't reply, Her excuse is simple. She never claimed conceited omnipotence. She has countless others clinging to her apron strings, including myriad species unable to speak for themselves. To Her elder offspring She says – 'Go raid the fridge. Go play outside. Go get a job. Or, better yet, lend me a hand. I have no time for idle whining.'" - David Brin, physicist and sci-fi writer

At a certain point, the rate of global extraction of crude petroleum products is reached, after which the rate of production enters a terminal decline. This is called "Peak Oil" and is another reason to become self-sustainable sooner than later. This is to say that there will come a day when our oil use will surpass the oil that's left in the ground, heading us towards the inevitable moment when there's no more left to power our cars and homes, our electric plants, to make our fertilizers and pesticides, or to run our farm equipment, or the trucks that bring us the food.

Let's talk again about how commercial farms work. A field is fertilized, and all commercial fertilizers are made from ammonium nitrate, which is made from natural gas. This is sprayed onto the fields by an oil-powered machine. Another oil-powered machine ploughs and another comes by and plants. The fields are irrigated with pumps powered by electricity, which comes from coal or, you guessed it: natural gas. But wait, there's more - oil-powered crop dusters spray oil-derived pesticides, once, twice, thrice. Then, when it's time to harvest, one oil-powered machine cuts, another loads, and another takes it to where it'll be processed by electric contraptions, and it's wrapped in plastic (made of oil) and trucked to a distribution center, then to the store. You can take it from there. There are 10 calories of hydrocarbon energy in every one calorie of food produced this way. Imagine that there's a finite amount of oil in the world and you'll soon realize that this would be a blatantly unsustainable system. Unfortunately, we'll soon be forced to see the end of this strategy.

Oil is made from the fossilized bodies of microorganisms, a process that takes millions of years. As of this writing, half of all the oil in the world has been used. The remaining half is of increasingly lower quality and will require more and more

> "Our agriculture system is almost wholly dependent on cheap fuel. Tremendous amounts of diesel fuel that are used in planting, and harvesting, and then, moving the stuff all these vast distances." - James Howard Kunstler *The Long Emergency*

energy to extract and refine. Oil is finite. Natural gas is finite, coal, uranium; all non-renewable energy sources are finite. There will be a peak for all of them. We're using, in a few decades, energy resources that took the planet millions of years to produce. Right now we are consuming 5 barrels of oil for every 1 barrel discovered.

For as long as I can remember, just about everyone I knew consumed like there was no tomorrow. My family threw away more food than many families in developing countries had. Now, when some of us in the West are just beginning to wake up to the realities of our wasteful lifestyle choices, those that have looked on hungrily for decades are starting to be able to enjoy the ease and luxury of modern life. In 1993, China had three quarters of a million cars on the road. At the start of 2004 they had 6 million, and now (2010) they have 24 million. The idea behind a "developing" country is that one day they'll be able to consume like a first world country; they'll be able to live like the people in the movies. But this is clearly impossible. Even Americans in the near future won't be able to consume like Americans today.

Most of us have our heads in the sand about this to one degree or another; we know there's a problem looming but we're hoping that if we bring our own bags to the supermarket it'll go away. But the average person in a developed country can't really be blamed; with the demands of modern life, most people are happy with just a few minutes a day to relax and enjoy the life they're working so hard for. We've never had a peak in resources before and we have blinders on about it. Like statistics about climate change or overpopulation on a piece of paper, it's not an idea we can easily digest. We need new role models.

Peak Oil Pioneers

From 1950 to 1990, Cuba lived comfortably under Soviet communist care. Then, with little warning in 1991, the Soviet Union collapsed and Cuba's access to oil dropped to less than 25%. Everything changed in a matter of weeks. Suddenly, malnourished children, anemic pregnant women, and underweight babies became commonplace. The impact on food production and availability was disastrous. The average Cuban lost 20 pounds. Massive blackouts made refrigeration difficult so the little food that was available would often spoil. Cubans had to wait 3 to 4 hours for a bus to take them to school or work, and when it came it was often full, so they'd have to wait another 3 to 4 for the next one. And when they finally got to work, there might be no power, or no materials for them to do their jobs.

Then in 1992, the 30-year-old American embargo of Cuba was tightened. Before, companies were prohibited from doing business with both communist Cuba and the freedom-defending USA. Now, any ship even docking in a Cuban port was denied access to the US for 6 months afterwards. Almost overnight, 750 million dollars worth of food and medical supplies pulled up anchor and sailed away.

"So we had now been like an experiment, with controlled conditions... Nothing, or very little... could get in from the outside, so everything had to happen from the inside. " - Roberto Perez, Cuban permaculturist and educator, from documentary film *The Power of Community*

Then in 1996, the stranglehold was intensified. Cuba abruptly found itself with almost no access to foreign resources. The American dollar was worth 150 pesos, and the average daily salary was worth 20 pesos. Cubans were making about 4 dollars a month, so money was no longer a commodity that could be used to acquire the basics of life. A recently comfortable society abruptly found itself cut-off, destitute, and hungry.

Every aspect of Cuban life was affected, but none more potently than farming. Before the collapse, Cuba's agriculture was more industrialized than any other Latin American country. It used a massive amount of fossil fuel for fertilizer, pesticides, farm machinery, and transportation - 2 or 3 times more than any other Latin American country, and acre for acre it surpassed the US in fertilizer consumption. Their farms had high yields, but these were in huge single-crop operations like tobacco, sugarcane, and citrus, which were exported while the basics were imported. The system wasn't set up to feed the people.

So the people: doctors, engineers, and lawyers, started sowing seeds in open places, without knowing how, because they were starving and there was no end in sight. The older generation, those that remembered how to operate a plough, how to tell if soil was acidic or alkaline by rolling it around in their mouths, were suddenly a valuable resource. A movement to use every arable piece of local land for growing food began. Every park, front yard, school, and vacant lot in Havana became a garden or orchard because there was no gas to transport food. And because there were no fossil fuels to produce chemical pesticides and fertilizers, over the months and seasons the fledgling farmers learned to use natural, organic pesticides like bugs and companion plants. Organic fertilizers like manure and compost were all they had.

They found ways to replenish the depleted soil with cheap and available resources, and to do their farming without the use of machinery. They used worms to turn sandy, dead soil into lush and nutrient-rich fertile ground. They found that they could extend the growing season by putting a fiber mesh between the plants and the sun, which would also control pests and was easily replaceable during hurricane season. As time went on, Cuban urban farmers found infinite small solutions to improve their lives. They dealt with the myriad complex problems that come with a new kind of agronomy by trial and error, and thrived. Formerly larger farms were divided up and leased to citizens for free by the government and the 2.2 million residents of Havana fed themselves from these rooftop gardens, schoolyard nurseries, and small farms within a few kilometers from the city.

Today, urban gardens in small Cuban cities and towns are even more productive, providing 80-100% of the residents' food, and over 80% of Cuba's food production is organic. In the 1980's, Cuba used 21,000 tons of chemical pesticides per year; now they use less than 1000. Good for the soil, good for the environment, good for the economy, and great for the people.

Now, apartment-dwellers with a well laid-out porch, rooftop, or patio garden improve their lives by both cutting back on their food-spending and selling their produce or homemade products like wine. Cuba's 140,000 urban farmers aren't the poorest people in society, as they are in many countries, like America, where farmers are constantly forced to cut corners and take the chemical way out. They are among the highest-paid professionals in the country, and are even exporting their natural pesticides, fertilizers, and knowledge to other countries. This rewarding occupation attracts people from all walks of life who don't want to be dependent on others for their sustenance. They have the respect of their communities and dignity of working in what has become one of the noblest professions.

The country as a whole is enjoying a slew of fringe benefits as well. They developed bio-organic farming methods because at the time they had no other choice. But now, with less than 2% of the population of Latin America, Cuba has 11% of its scientists. At the start of the "Special Period", the name for Cuba's quiet revolution starting with the collapse of the Soviet Union, Cuba had

"It wasn't the *Exxon Valdez* captain's driving that caused the Alaskan oil spill. It was yours." - Greenpeace advertisement, 1990

3 universities. It now has about 50, with 7 in Havana alone. Cuba's urban farmers produce much more from the same amount of land than their corporate counterparts, and many of them donate a portion of their crops to the elderly, day-care centers and schools, orphanages, and pregnant women. They do this for free with no government involvement, because they want their community to thrive. Small farmers form co-ops, if they wish, to buy in bulk and share machinery. In many cities in richer countries, we don't even *know* our neighbors.

Cuba has roughly the same life expectancy and infant mortality rate as the US, though the average citizen uses 1/8th the energy and resources of the average American. They were once forced to be frugal with their energy consumption, using the sun to pre-heat cooking water, for example, but now it's a way of life. Why do most American homes have their hot-water heaters in cold closets and basements, requiring more fossil fuels to heat them, instead of outside in the sun? Sugar mills, which produce gas when the fibers are heated, are used as power plants, which now provide the country with 30% of its energy during harvest seasons. Increased walking and biking improved Cubans' fitness and drastically reduced diabetes (51% less deaths attributed to diabetes since before the Soviet collapse), heart disease (35% less), and strokes (20% less, and 18% less deaths overall). Cuba trains more doctors than they need, more than double the number of physician-to-citizen ration as America, and sends the surplus to developing countries around the world. Urban planners from all over the world study Havana as a model of livability. 85% of Cubans own their own home. The countryside, which has been called the last romantic place on earth, looks like a science-fiction comic book come alive with solar cell home-spun shacks, country school and rural hospitals. Cuba has reclaimed its health, its communities, its ethos, and its future.

The fact that Cuba is still looking for oil off their shores may surprise some. But unlike the vampires in developed countries that will start wars and enslave weaker nations for the life-blood of their consumer culture, they don't use what they find. If Cuba does hit upon the Texas tea, they sell it to wealthier countries at a premium, because they know how to get by without it. We can wait until our own energy crisis to enact sustainable practices, and certainly the GOP government and their "head in the sand" policy-making will wait until it's too late, or we can make changes now while we have some breathing room.

The concept of peak oil brings up another, much bigger question: what will happen to us when the greasy lubricant of our society becomes too expensive to be a viable means of energy?

Easter Island's Last Lumberjack

Easter Island is a remote dot of earth about 1500 miles off the coast of Chile. It's so small you can walk around the whole thing in a day. It's also the hauntingly desolate remains of a once-thriving civilization that numbered over 10,000 people.

When Easter Island was settled by 20 or 30 Polynesians halfway through the first millennium, it was a lush forest. The sweet

"There is a sufficiency in the world for man's need but not for man's greed." – Mahatma Gandhi

potatoes and other crops the settlers brought with them thrived in the rich soil, living was easy, and the Easter Islanders found themselves with lots of free time. In about 1000 years, they swelled to a burgeoning society, and one of the most technologically advanced in the ancient world. Crops were protected by complex rock formations, and by some accounts every rock on the island was moved at least 3 or 4 times. The island's famous 600 stone statues, many of which were in sophisticated astronomical alignment, weighed tens of tons and were transported by human force, often for several miles over forested, hilly terrain. Each monument was laboriously carved from different color rock from quarries all over the island so the leaders of the clans could ask for favors from the Gods, and for a while it seemed to be working. But when European explorers reached the island in 1722, they found an arid grassland with less than 2000 malnourished people, many of who had become cannibals, living in squalid reed huts and constant warfare. The explorers couldn't fathom how such a primitive society could be responsible for the socially and technologically advanced monuments, and because the island was now a barren prairie, the transportation of behemoth idols seemed impossible. When asked how the 20-foot-high stone gods had gotten there, the inhabitants, wholly disconnected from their history, replied simply, "They walked".

Actually, the statues were pushed along rolling roads made of the island's trees, chopped down in huge swathes to make way for the huge stone carvings and laid side-by-side through miles of forest. The trees, which provided shelter, canoes for fishing, and fuel, were so abundant at the time that they could be used without fear of running out. But as the population continued to swell, and more and more clans were formed with more leaders, all needed their own statues lest their dependants miss out on their slice of the divine benevolence pie and the ability to live as well as their neighbors. Competition for resources between clans grew fierce, and then someone, one day, cut down the last tree on the island. No more boats for fishing. No more fuel for heat, cooking, or transporting statues. The topsoil eroded at a breakneck pace and the gravely land couldn't hold in moisture or nutrients. Hundreds of great stone deities were abandoned, unfinished, in quarries around the islands. The gods were not happy. With no logs for buildings, people began living in caves and flimsy reed huts, fiercely protecting their meager assets. Cannibalism became a reasonable means of dealing with both enemies and hunger. Like the Romans, Byzantines, Vikings, and Mayans before them, the Easter Islanders didn't think total collapse could happen to them, and lived recklessly until it did.

The pattern is clear. When civilizations over-consume, they cut off the legs of their own life-support systems and begin to fight each other over what little is left. Then they either starve or leave. Our current problems are global: climate change, overpopulation, peak oil, genetically manipulated genes out-crossing into the DNA of the world's food supply; so there's nowhere to go, just like boatless Easter Islanders on a remote island in the middle of the Pacific. We can't abandon our planet and set off for a new Eden. We're here, and we have only two choices: cut down the last tree, or take an objective look at the dilemmas facing our species as a whole, and find another way to live.

> "We never know the worth of water till the well is dry." - Thomas Fuller, *Gnomologia*, 1732

A very early action of the Bush administration upon assuming office in 2001 was to lobby for the replacement of the chairman of the official United Nations Intergovernmental Panel on Climate Change (IPCC). This was done at the request of Exxon, who felt the sitting chairman, Dr. Watson, was too "aggressive" in pursuing action on the issue of global warming. As a result of actions taken by the administration, Dr. Watson was replaced ("at the request of the US") by the industry-friendly Dr.

Rajendra Pachauri, hand-picked by the administration, and referred to by former vice-president Al Gore as the "let's drag our feet" candidate. Four years later, Dr. Pachauri issued the strongest warning yet in regard to global climate change, and a most urgent call for immediate action. His report stated that there is not a moment to lose, and added that we are risking the ability of the human race to survive. He called for "very deep" cuts in current pollution levels, stating that the point of no return was rapidly approaching.

"The American way of life is non-negotiable" - Dick Cheney

Sometimes big change comes through a big effort. But more often, revolution is the result of very small actions repeated over time. For a while, maybe for several generations, the results of our efforts are almost unnoticeable, but then there comes a "tipping point" where the slow incremental change has completely reshaped society. It's like driving. Turn the wheel dramatically and you find yourself on the beginning of a different road, or in a ditch. But turn the wheel just 5 degrees, and for a while it seems like nothing's different. Then, after enough miles, the car is in a completely different place, a totally different course. This is the way to lasting change, to guaranteed metamorphosis. When someone wants a major turn-around in their health, for example, I always recommend making one small change a day. In a year, they'll have made 365 little improvements, which adds up to a big difference. And they'll have made new habits and the stamina to maintain them, encouraged by the changes they notice in their life, how they feel, etc. I encourage treating anything important as a marathon, not a sprint, and digging in for the long haul.

It's true that massive change is overdue: in the way we treat each other, our world, and ourselves. But I don't have the dynamite, nor a flair for drama. Instead, I just make one improvement at a time, stabilize it, and then see where I'm at. I've gotten excited and gung-ho about a lot of things in my life, but I've noticed that permanent and powerful transformation has come about from a sustained 5% turn of the wheel. If you're different, that's awesome, together I hope we can make something really magical happen.

"Greater than the tread of mighty armies is *an idea whose time has come.*" - Victor Hugo

Everyone but the Kitchen Sink: Modernization, McDonald's, and Hyper-Maturation

I'd like to make it clear that this book is for absolutely everyone. The ways of making and preparing food in here aren't just for already-organic urban yoga hipster families; they're for the low-income families that can't afford fresh vegetables, communities and aid-workers in developing countries, and the one-third of American kids that eat fast food every day.

Evolution is slow; it certainly can't keep up with the modernization of our diets. Our Paleolithic hunter-gatherer ancestors lived on hundreds of different wild plant sources, some meat (in the few climates where killing a creature that was running or fighting for its life was less effort than foraging for edible plants), and thereby guaranteed themselves a vast array of potent, living nutrients. Just to put it in perspective, of the food crops grown in 1900, 97% were extinct in 2000, just a hundred years later. And we're talking about the vast changes in lifestyle over the course of half a million years, while our basic biology has stayed the same. In the prehistoric world, starch, fat, and salt were rare commodities that our brains were programmed to seek out with the fervor of junkies. Now, they are available on every street corner in the developed world, and the fast food "restaurants" that offer them claim different characteristics and even different cultures. Starch, fat, and salt are found in almost every case in the precise proportions that mirror the cravings imprinted in our very genes, with lab-concocted cocktails of smells pumped into the air to lure our Paleolithic minds in the door.

Ten thousand years ago (a time frame too short to cause many genetic changes, though one exception is the continued production of lactase, the milk enzyme, in about 25% of post-nursing humans), our ancestors went from a wild food diet totally free of grains to an agricultural lifestyle, in a move that author and UCLA Professor of Physiology Dr. Jared Diamond calls "The Worst Mistake in the History of the Human Race", in his essay of the same name. Our forefathers began growing not the crops that would protect the delicate balance of their health and longevity, but the ones that were the easiest to cultivate, harvest, and store: wheat, rice, and corn began providing the most calories to humanity. The average lifespan promptly dropped seven years[2].

It's no surprise that we're not cut out for the amount of starch, salt and particularly fat in our diet, as it's quickly killing us; heart disease, diabetes, and cancer are all linked to a diet too high in these foods. McDonalds lost two CEOs in a single year to diet-related diseases (2004): heart attack and colon cancer[3]. The majority of Americans are on at least one prescription drug to treat type-2 diabetes, cholesterol, and high blood pressure, all of which are directly related to starch, fat, or salt.

Less lethal but just as alarming are the effects of diets high in trans- and saturated fats on children. The number of overweight children has tripled in the last three decades. Kids' menus at sit-down restaurants are usually much worse than the adults'. Our schools are "7-11's with books" (Yale diet expert Kelly Brownell). Shortened and less happy lives will be the obvious result, but there are more nefarious effects as well. Throughout most of our species' history, female sexual maturity was reached at 17 ½ to 18 years old. In 1900, the age had dropped to 15 ½ in developed countries, and now the average age that girls reach puberty is 11, while many girls mature sexually at 9 or 10. Many researchers originally believed this accelerating change was due to ingesting the hormones

---

[2] Pia Bennike, *Paleopathology of Danish Skeletons* [Copenhagen: Almquist and Wiskell, 1985]; and N-G Gejvall, *Westerhu: Medeviel Populations and Church in the Light of Skeletal Remains* [Lund: Hakan Ohlssons Boktryckeri, 1960]

[3] I'd like to add, however, that the second CEO, Australian Charlie Bell, perhaps prompted by the release of the documentary film Super Size Me criticizing the health of McDonald's food, led efforts to add healthier choices to the McDonald's menu and offered parents the option to substitute juice and apple slices for fries and soft drinks for their children. The "Supersize" option was also eliminated.

given to milk cows and meat animals to speed *their* maturation and growth, but recent studies show that the single greatest cause is the estrogenic effect of additional fat cells in the girls' bodies. Boys show a much less dramatic change, putting them far out of sync with the girls, with the exception of the most overweight boys whose puberty is actually slowed down by the increased estrogen in their body fat. One result of living out of harmony with our biology.

Cultural awareness of the alarming health problems has been steadily growing over the past decade. Ten years ago the public acknowledged that we were in the throes of a losing battle with obesity and heart disease. Two-thirds of Americans were overweight. Obesity-related illnesses killed a third of a million people every year, crippling millions, and costing our health care system almost a hundred billion dollars annually. Overwhelmingly, people singled out their excess weight as the thing they most disliked about their bodies.

In the past ten years, Americans have made a number of choices about their diet and health. The average American has eaten 50% *more* fast food meals and 5 more pounds of sugar per year. Hospital bills related to obesity have risen to $117 billion, and it's estimated that 8 out of 10 Americans are or will become overweight.

In 2004, the World Health Organization proposed dietary guidelines to reduce fat and sugar consumption. The US delegation, which represents the fattest nation in the world, protested these changes, on behalf of the food industry, as "scientifically unproven". While the WHO guidelines call on governments to reduce the unhealthy food advertising aimed at children and use fiscal incentives to limit the availability of junk food and amount of trans fats in the diet, the US Department of Health and Human Services responded that it would be best to use tactics like "better data and surveillance, and the promotion of sustainable strategies that focus on energy balance," hollow and meaningless expressions with just enough buzzwords to dupe the most foolish into thinking that something was being done.

Former senator Peter Fitzgerald noted that putting the USDA, whose first job it is to sell agricultural products, in charge of our dietary guidelines was like "putting a fox in charge of the hen house". The USDA subsidizes farmers to grow high-calorie, low nutrition crops for $19 billion annually, making white flour, corn syrup, hydrogenated margarine, and white rice cost sometimes less than nothing to produce. It becomes these foods that are the most heavily-advertised and make up the bulk of ingredients of fast food, junk food, and school lunches. And while the current administration is offering small subsidies to farms that convert to organic methods, an initiative spearheaded by Mrs. Obama (who is taking much of the ill-placed heat from farmers losing their hard-won handouts), still not a penny goes towards large-scale vegetable farming. I've gone into such detail in these last few paragraphs to illuminate the fact that the very government agencies we've put in place to protect our health and well-being can't be counted on to do that very thing. It is, once again, up to us to take responsibility for our own health.

But it's difficult to choose fresh food when $5 feeds a busy family at McDonald's. Fast and junk food are designed to maximize the cheapest ingredients, and grocery stores can rarely compete. Add to that the time it takes to shop for and prepare dinner and it becomes a daunting task for haggard parents. But an even less expensive meal, both in money and in medical bills, can be had with a deep breath, a few minutes' forethought, and the application of the methods in this book, in even less time than it takes to round up the kids and drive to the transfat pusher on the corner with a winning goatee and bowtie or cute red pigtails. While the dangers of not making a change in our families' diets could be their own encyclopedia, the benefits of doing so are simple: turning our children into vivacious young people with strong immune systems, increased focus and learning - the kids they were meant to be. It's my fervent desire that the mostly unoriginal ideas presented in these books will spread not only to the families that can most easily implement them, but also to the ones that need them most.

Changing Food Habits - Using the Brain for a Change

I doubt that the previous section is enough to shock people into changing their diets. We all know what to do to be healthier: eat more vegetables and less crap, exercise. It's usually not the why nor the what that holds us up, but the how. Willpower or self-talk alone isn't enough to make lasting changes for most people, and just like the force that drives us to continue eating the ice cream our conscious minds know we've had enough of, the reason is our wiring.

The human brain is "an organ so complex we may never fully understand it", says Colin Blakemore, British neurobiologist. There are 100 billion nerve cells in the brain, with ten thousand times as many connections between them. On average, our brains make one million data transfers every second, for the entirety of our lifetimes. Recent studies have found brain cells previously thought to exist only inside our skulls are actually dispersed throughout our entire bodies, amplifying the previous number by orders of magnitude.

In addition to being the miraculous instrument of human achievement, according to David Linden, a professor of neuroscience at Johns Hopkins University, the brain is a "cobbled-together mess... quirky, inefficient and bizarre ... a weird agglomeration of ad hoc solutions that have accumulated throughout millions of years of evolutionary history," he states in his book, "The Accidental Mind," from Harvard University Press. Interestingly, when new kingdoms of species evolved: reptiles to mammals, lower mammals to humans, the brain didn't actually evolve. The entire reptilian brain stayed almost as is, and a new brain was added on top. That means that we're all carrying around the brains of a flatworm, a snake and a primate right next to our advanced thinking capabilities.

The reptilian area of the brain governs habits and emotions and will always choose the easy route if left to its own, literally subconscious, devices. Specifically, the basal ganglia (BG) is a loosely grouped collection of nerve cells located deep within the reptilian part of each cerebral hemisphere. It's responsible for rage, fear, love, lust, contentment, and automatic behaviors like slamming on the brakes, smashing a vase against a wall in startling anger, or opening the fridge to grab the cheesecake before you even know you're doing it. The pre-frontal cortex (PFC) is the newest addition to the human brain, situated right behind the forehead and is in charge of the things that make us human: personality and executive functions: goal-setting, understanding consequences, and differentiating between conflicting thoughts to choose (hopefully) the most enlightened course of action. Basically, it's considered to be the conscious conductor in the orchestration of thoughts and actions in accordance with internal goals. The BG pushes for habitual behavior, while the PFC considers whether or not that deed is going to bring us what we want in the long run. An over-simplified example of this is the drug-addicted brain, which tells the owner in increasingly creative ways that more drugs are needed. We know as observers that the best course of action is to re-shape the desires of the BG by stopping the drug use and consequently changing the messages being sent to the PFC, but just like an addict's brain invents evidence to show that more drug use is the best course of action, within the individual an entirely different story is told.

An iguana or python doesn't respond to coaxing, cajoling, or bargaining; it changes its habits based on repetition, pure and simple. The ritualistic nature of this organ leaves no room for complex emotions (my apologies to the shirtless-under-their-leather-vests guys at the beach with their scaly loved ones.) The time it takes to change a habit depends on how ingrained it is. It's a simple formula. When a wagon wheel goes over the same road, in the same way, an ever-deepening rut results. If the wheel happens to find new ground, all it takes is a little push in the same old direction and the wheel teeters then returns to the rut. But push in a new direction everyday and the wheel will in no time make a new groove, soon becoming deeper than the first and the wheel will easily stay into it, propelling the cart effortlessly in a new direction. Absolutely any habit can change from a rut to a groove, given enough pushes. Research states that simple habits take 21 days to break, and while we're dealing with more complicated lifestyle changes, 3 weeks of daily action and at least the beginnings of changes are guaranteed. If it's a worthwhile goal, these incremental encouragements may, like signposts on the proverbial road, be all that's needed to propel you towards lasting change. It all starts with one action, today.

The pleasure mechanism in the human brain is *extremely*

flexible. It will attach to whatever is introduced, whether unconsciously, like heroin or Big Macs, or consciously like whole living foods. We can quite literally re-engineer our evolution, rewire our brains. The brain of someone who has made a habit of a simple sprout salad with homemade vinaigrette will release just as much dopamine, the "pleasure chemical", as a steak and potatoes guy will get from his 20-oz ribeye. The satisfaction of improving our health and the self-esteem that results is enough to pull back the veil of denial that results in actions that destroy ourselves, other creatures, and the planet, and we will soon have a network of habits and beliefs that will make it easy for us to make better choices.

I know from personal experience. As I slowly started eating more and more whole, living, simple foods, I was surprised to find myself craving whole, living, simple foods. If you've never jones-ed after raw baby spinach, it is a pretty wonderful feeling. Processed food started looking like wax fruit, (e.g. - not food), and non-organic food had an unmistakably flat and empty taste. When I travel, I try to sprout as much food as possible and I obviously lean towards authentic and clean cuisines, especially in places like Germany where GMOs are outlawed and almost all the food is grown with traditional organic methods. It's not always possible or polite to eat this way, however, and after a month or two of bratwurst, potato salad, and strudel and the impulses coming from my BG have become quite distorted. It takes just a few meals to start affecting unconstructive change, and about 3-4 times as long to re-position positive habits in the BG. I don't know why negative transformation seems to have more pull than the other direction, but when I get back home I'm bolstered by the fact that the challenging choices I face will soon become effortless, and because of the nature of the basal ganglia-pre-frontal cortex connection, dramatic changes in behavior can make it even easier. Humans have the largest PFC of any animal. Let's put it to use for a better life now and a brighter future for the planet.

Transitioning to a Living Diet

When we're used to cooked food, we usually look for one thing out of our meals, besides the immediate taste sensations: a "feeling of fullness". Living foods nourish our bodies in a completely different, and much more thorough way. This became clear to me during a recent dinner I prepared for some friends and family where one person refused to eat the meal, worrying that they were sure they "wouldn't get filled up from it". That relation grabbed a sandwich from a nearby convenience store and scarfed the fistful of spongy white bread and deli meats while the rest of us enjoyed a living meal. Afterwards, I noticed the general ebullience of the family and the heavy, lethargic quality of that individual. Granted, their food choice may have been healthier if they hadn't had to scrounge for dinner after being ambushed by an alfalfa-wielding hippie, but it's an interesting dichotomy. The "fill your belly", "stick to your ribs" mentality is quite the opposite of being fed on a cellular level, really nourished down to the nerve, where the energy that used to go into digestion and assimilation are already in the food and don't need to be stolen from the body's other processes. It's a different kind of satisfaction with living food when you're used to heavy meats and caramelized starches, but in time you will adjust, if you choose to go that route.

Table 2: Seed/Nut Digestibility Chart

How	What	Why
Toasted	Starches (usually the main component) are caramelized and impossible to utilize. Most vitamins and minerals diminished or gone. Enzymes gone. Some oils are toxic.	Enzymes are destroyed over 108 degrees; most nutrients are destroyed at high temperatures. Heating some oils past 170 degrees creates free radicals and other toxins.1
Raw, right outta the bag	The most difficult to digest and assimilate; heating does destroy (denature the molecular bonds and render inert) some EI's.	Nutrients are in a dormant state and bound with EI's; these rob the body of its own enzymes and more effort than necessary is put into digestion, while less energy than possible is gotten out in nutrition. The living enzymes of the seed are dormant and unusable.
Soaked in water	Easier to handle, but not at peak nutrition.	Soaking starts the germination process, breaking down the EI's so they can be rinsed

		away, but enzymes aren't fully activated, nor are nutrient levels substantially increased, but you're on the right track...
Fermented (in probiotic water, miso, or seed cheese, for example)	Partial probiotic pre-digestion makes protein, healthy fats, vitamins, minerals, and starches present in dormant seed more available.	Beneficial microorganisms go to work on the starches and long-chain proteins, turning them into more easily-digestible simple sugars and amino acids, and thereby taking some of the strain off of the human. Blending with probiotic water releases EI's which are removed by bacteria.
Sprouted	Nutrient levels are at their peak, enzymes fully active. Provides the body with the building blocks of health and an abundance of energy with	

	which to use them.	
Sprouted and Fermented	Bacteria make immunity-supporting compounds you can't get anywhere else. Peak nutrition and complex components broken down into easily-assimilable forms. The benefits of the seed's inherent nutrition and life force, the short-term benevolent action of friendly bacteria on the seed and the long-term advantages to the digestive system as probiotics settle in and prepare to convert everything that comes their way into a greater you.	Plus it tastes freaking awesome.

The "How?"

Fermenting

This chapter won't teach you how to make more food for less dough like the ones on sprouting and growing will, but you will learn how to make the food you have more nutritious, digestible, interesting, and last a whole lot longer. Fermented foods also have longer-lasting health benefits, as the beneficial bacteria you'll be cultivating will devotedly colonize your digestive system and, given the right conditions, can continue to enthusiastically propagate for the rest of your life.

Fermentation is what happens when microorganisms 1) digest sugar,

> "Bacteria keep us from heaven and put us there." - Martin H. Fischer, 19th-century physician and writer

whether from cane, fruit, dairy, or starch, turning it into new and beneficial compounds, and 2) break the bonds of hardy molecules into their easier-to-digest, simpler components. This healthful process changes the nature of food and drink, giving us cheese, sauerkraut, yogurt, beer, soda, and countless other new and wonderful foods that come from all around the world. Home growing and sprouting is a significant way to take control of your health, but fermentation, though cheap and easy, is just as important.

A Brief History of Slime

For as long as humans have been on the planet, fermented foods have been appreciated for their distinctive flavors and nutritional benefits. They have sustained people through long winters and sea voyages, frequently and dramatically changed the course of human history, and their creation has been attributed to the gods. The real agents in the mystical transformation of honey into intoxicating nectar, cabbage into sauerkraut, grapejuice into wine, and cyanide-laden tubers into nutritious food that sustains the native peoples of Central America, are the oldest, wisest, and most mysterious life forms on the planet.

> "Bacteria have studied us more closely and more lovingly than any other creature. Even your dog can't give you the devotion that bacteria do." - Abigail Salyers, Ph. D, Professor of Microbiology at the University of Illinois.

Microorganisms, recognized for their health-giving benefits since the end of the 19th century, were thought to battle the disease-causing putrefaction of foods in the human digestive system. They are, of course, also responsible for said fermentation, but though ye olde scientists were wrong about the source of disease, they were onto something about the pro-biotic (good-for-life) potential of some of those unseen beings. In the two centuries since, beneficial single-celled organisms have been recognized not only as guards against pathogens but also as intelligent collaborators without whom life, and certainly vibrant health, would be absolutely impossible. Many people are surprised to hear that bacteria make up 10% of our body weight, and the percentages of those organisms that are helpful, neutral, or harmful is mainly the result of lifestyle choices. Even more surprising is that 90% of the cells in our body are bacterial cells, so only 10% of the cells in our bodies are actually human cells, "us" by the common mode of thinking. (The discrepancy in those two percentages, you clever rabbits, is due to the varying size of cells, microbes being very small and animal cells being very large.) In fact, it's a common expression in the bacteriological world that "we're just a colony of bacteria carrying around a little bit of person." A good reason to find out what microscopic organisms are all about.

"Support bacteria - they're the only culture some people have." - Stephen Wright

DNA Sluts and Your Guts: *Genetic Promiscuity* and its effect on human evolution and happiness

An amazing behavior of microorganisms hints that the evolutionary enlightenment of the quadrillion (that a 1 with 15 zeros) little buddies we are hosting in and on our bodies ("we" and "hosting" have already been shown to be meaningless words, but we'll stay in the point of view of humans, for now) may have a lot more to do with the quality of our lives than whether or not we're constipated.

Bacteria have a strange and extremely effective way of learning. They share their experiences with any microbe who'll listen, and learn what their billions of neighbors know just by making a little cell-to-cell contact. They do this by something bacteriologists (and now you!) call "parallel gene transfer", or genetic promiscuity. This is the process whereby bacteria can exchange pieces of their DNA with neighboring organisms right through their cell membranes whenever they're in contact, just like plugging your ipod into a friend's computer. What's even more surprising is that they don't distinguish who they share with, even passing new traits, like how to resist new antibiotic drugs, between species, those naughty little critters. This is how they've been able to evolve so quickly into the incredibly efficient examples of evolution they are. When I say quickly, I'm talking about 4 billion years of evolution, each minute of which they've used with superlative efficiency.

Human DNA is a few tens of thousands of genes, compressed into the nucleus of our cells, which contain the codes for every part of our body, from the color of our eyes to the shape of the tiny connective tissues in our little toes, as well as many of our personality traits, as shown by studies of identical twins adopted by different families. Only 2%-3% of this information codes for proteins, so modern science calls the rest "junk DNA" (though some scientists feel that non-coding DNA might be more important than the rest.) Bacterial cells, on the other hand, are wall-to-wall DNA, containing 300 times more genes than humans. And they have only *one* cell to blueprint.

This fact alone (and there are many, many others) proves that they, not us whose laborious evolution happens not every few minutes like bacteria, but every 20 or so years, are the epitome of evolution. So when a bacterium develops a resistance to a certain antibiotic in Paris, for example, bacteria all over the world will have the same inside information in a matter of *hours*. This is only one way microbes communicate and probably not the most fantastical, considering new research which shows that some bacteria can also conduct electricity, sharing news by zapping their neighbors with charged electrons imprinted with data. Or that "magnetotactic" bacteria DNA create organs that contain magnetic crystals, which, sensitive to the Earth's magnetic field, tell a bacterium where it is on an unimaginably vast planet. We think of microbes living out their insentient lives in a square centimeter of soil or floating along aimlessly in a drop of water; why would a microscopic organism need a GPS? So when you consider the fact that "you" are 9/10ths bacteria, and that most of the other 1/10th of your cells are very recently *evolved* from bacterial cells, the nature of those organisms seems a matter too important to leave to chance or superstition.

Public Enemy #1: The War on Bugs

In ancient times, the Egyptians, Chinese, and Natives of Central America, and other primitive cultures used molds to combat infections, presumably without understanding the antibacterial property of mold and its connection to the treatment of disease. It wasn't until the turn of the 19th century that the surgeon Joseph Lister noticed that urine contaminated with mold wouldn't allow bacteria to grow freely.

In 1928, the world of disease-causing bacteria was checkmated when Alexander Fleming, a bacteriologist working at St. Mary's Hospital in London, observed that a petri dish of staphylococcus had been contaminated with a blue-green mold and that cultures of the bacteria adjacent to the mold were dissolving. Studies confirmed that this "penicillin" would be humanity's first and final weapon against sickness, Nobel prizes were awarded, and large-scale production was begun. Antibiotics, from the Greek "against-life", would ease suffering, save countless lives, and make the Earth more sanitary for all.

Then, only a year later, there was a problem. Strains of bacteria began popping up in hospitals that wouldn't bat a microscopic eye at penicillin. They had developed "resistance" to that weapon, and stronger tools became necessary. So steady-handed early-1940's biologists began coming up with more powerful antibiotics that would take final care of these misfit microorganisms, and attempted to strike the delicate balance between strong enough to kill the bacteria but not so strong that they would kill the patient. They sometimes succeeded. And so began the war *with* drugs that rages on to this day.

As discussed above, while humans like to think that they're highly evolved compared to microorganisms and therefore the "pages" making up the book of our DNA are also more advanced, but in fact the opposite is true. There are no wasted letters or no wasted space in their genes, which are essentially wall-to-wall

"This body ain't big enough for the both of us". - Bacterium Bill

efficient data. Bacteria have become perfect machines of function and evolution. These are the unseen "cultures" we've decided to do battle upon, so that now, in our weakened state, debilitated by the slightest contact with a pathogen, we have no choice but to soldier on in the fight.

And this is a war that science is losing. "In several member states between 25 per cent and more than 60 per cent of bloodstream infections caused by one type of pneumonia bug were found to have combined resistance to multiple antibiotics", the ECDC [European Centre for Disease Control] said.

"For the patients who are infected with these bacteria, few last-line antibiotics ... remain available," said Marc Sprenger, the ECDC's director.[4] He's referring mainly to thanklemesien, the nuclear bomb antibiotic – physician's last-ditch effort against the super-bugs popping up everywhere from Berlin to New Delhi.

"The sheer tonnage of antibiotics that [are] used in the world every year… contributes to the problem of resistant bacteria in the community, which then becomes a problem in the hospital… I can't think of a microbiologist that would say that the wide application of antibiotics will do anything but select for antibiotic-resistant organisms. That's a consequence of… strains that won't be resistant to that antibiotic in the future." Michael Scheld. M.D., Professor of Surgery, University of Virginia Health Sciences Center

4
grows" Reuters London News Release ABP.

Even so, over 18 million antibiotic prescriptions were written last year for colds, which are caused by viruses, and *not* bacteria. It seems obvious, based on this track record, that we'll soon be out of options. In fact, a Tokyo patient recently died due to a thanklemesien-resistant strain of staphylococcus. A microorganism that, with all my sympathies and condolences to the families of people that have lost the battle with this infection, is easily overcome by a strong immune system.

It was in fact, Louis Pasteur himself, who first discovered how to kill microorganisms with heat by a technique named after him, who said: "It's the microbes that will have the last word."

Bacteria, microorganisms, probiotics, microflora – whether scary or sought after, these little critters make our existence possible. They're intimately involved with our birth, death, first meal and our last one, and pretty much everything that happens in between.

> "Science is the first word on everything, and the last word on nothing" – Victor Hugo

Your First Fermentation: Probiotic Water

The easiest and cheapest way to supplement with beneficial organisms is "probiotic water". This recipe makes use of fresh grain or seed sprouts to invite advantageous microflora to gently ferment water, which we can (and should) drink every day. It can also be a potent starter for other fermentations, like seed cheese.

Probiotic water (called "rejuvelac" by the old-timers) is very simple to make. It's a two-step process, the first is something you already know how to do from Volume 1 of Kitchen Sink Farming: Sprouting. First, seeds are sprouted (grains from the wheat family make the most popular flavor, though it can be made with any sprouted seed), then they're thrown into water and left to brew for a day or two. Some o' them old timers also talk about what grains make the "most nutritious rejuvelac", but this is an unnecessary occupation. Because the seeds don't have to be eaten, only the liquid used, taste is the only consideration, so experiment. Wheat is the most popular because of its yeasty-lemony flavor, and spelt, with its buttery quality, makes a slightly effervescent, cloudy tonic like I imagine Harry Potter's butterbeer to be. Rye's flavor translates nicely as a probiotic water, and the addition of some sprouted fennel or caraway seeds will take the imbiber back to their childhood among New York's Jewish delis, whether or not they had one. These are all great on their own as delicious health tonics and digestive aids, but the culinary possibilities are quite limitless, such as a base for tomato soup with a hint of pickle and pumpernickel, or a red-lentil marinara with the divine sparkle of life.

Probiotic water is rife with lactobacillus bacteria like acidophilus and bifidus and is a great alternative to store-bought probiotics. Homemade probiotics take just minutes of effort to brew over the course of a week, from seed to sprout to sip, are more potent and, as I once found while looking at an opened capsule of acidophilus next to a drop of probiotic water under my microscope, are about 40,000 times cheaper. Additionally, I've tried a few times to make "designer" probiotics, that is, to use those expensive, name-brand flora to start a little culture of home flora, and wouldn't you know it, those ridiculously expensive little pills of bacteria would always go bad in the relatively gentle environment of my home-made probiotic water. Either the bacteria in my kitchen are a super-strength strain, or a fresh, living, lovingly-cultivated culture is unrivaled in vitality and potency to lab-grown, cryogenically frozen bacteria stagnating in bottles on supermarket shelves.

The recipe is as follows:

1 Cup Dry Seed or Grain

Sprout in a jar with a screen on top in the normal fashion (See Kitchen Sink Farming Vol. 1: Sprouting. Or, google it).

When the seeds have been growing tails for a day or two (not just poked out, but not longer than the seed itself), either rinse them one last time or don't. The reason FOR rinsing them would be to remove the last bit of enzyme inhibitors that are clinging to them; the reason for NOT rinsing is to leave be the probiotics that have slipped in and settled. The first depends on what seed you're using: soybeans and quinoa could use an extra rinse, and the second is determined by strength of the flora in your local environment. Have you been culturing for months or years? Then cleaner is probably better. Is this your first ferment in a Manhattan high-rise? Then you should probably treat your microbes with kid gloves. It's a fairly unimportant difference and I'm sure you'll be fine either way, but if you're nerdy by nature like me, now you know.

Fill the jar with pure water (now you know why we used a jar. You don't even need to take off the screen) and set it somewhere warm, clean and dark, with good air circulation. If you have small bugs around, you can replace the screen with a cloth. The top of a refrigerator or in a warm cabinet with the door ajar work nicely - it will ferment more quickly in a warmer, moist environment. Leave it for 24 hours, then taste it. If it tastes like water, leave it for another day. We're looking for a lightly sour, pleasant taste; if the taste is too much, toss it and start over. One of the benefits of that 1:40,000 dollar ratio.

Probiotic water is a delicate, largely unprotected brew and there will be a point where unhelpful "bad" bacteria will move in and take over. This will be characterized by an increasingly foul smell and flavor; and we obviously want to stop the fermentation before that, while still cultivating the most numerous beneficial bacteria.

When the brew is at its peak, screw a lid on the jar and put the whole thing in the fridge, or you may want to strain just the liquid into a bottle for two reasons: 1) to take up less room in the fridge, or 2) to immediately start another batch of brew using new water and the same sprouts. The sprouted grains or seeds are generally good for two batches; after that they tend to start floating to the surface and attracting unfriendly bacteria. Putting an active fermentation in the refrigerator is called *cold stabilization* by wine geeks and thick-bearded home brewers, and refers to the fact that bacteria slow way down in the cold and stabilize their metabolic processes – fermentation pretty much stops. A half-day in the warmth of the world equals a week or two in the refrigerator. Your probiotic water is ready to be drunk straight, used in food preparation, or used to start other fermentations, and the sprouted seeds can be tossed, or (preferably) used as more flavorful versions of their unfermented selves.

Recap:

Sprout 1 cup of any seed or grain with the jar method.

When the tail is as long as the seed, fill the jar with water, leaving the screen on, and place in a dark, temperate place.

In 2-3 days, put it in the fridge, or strain out the probiotic water (putting that in the fridge) and cover the sprouts with new water, fermenting once more.

Local Flora

Sauerkrauts and other fermented veggies

As we've discussed, bacteria are everywhere on Earth, from the cold and lifeless ocean depths to the upper stratosphere, where powerful ultra-violet light exists that would instantly vaporize a less adaptive organism. Thriving in the boiling geysers of Yosemite, active volcanoes, and nuclear reactors, bacteria effortlessly colonize every surface of your kitchen. On your skin, in your digestive tract, and within your very blood they flourish, and no amount of scrubbing with anti-bacterial soap is going to change that. And why would we want it to? Bacteria have been here long before us, preparing the world for our presence in a myriad of ways, and will be here long after us, whatever the reason for our demise.

Enough time has passed, I suppose, from the sanitation craze of the 50's that extended past countertops into relationships and politics, though never as thoroughly as we were led to believe. Now many people accept the benefits of probiotics in neat little capsules or yogurt, much of which has been ungratefully re-pasteurized; once the lactobacilli have served their intended purpose they're warily cooked up under watchful, darkly circled eyes. There's even a growing market for raw milk products, whose microbial populations remain intact along with the natural compounds, usually boiled away or uselessly caramelized, that allow the benefits of milk, so noisily marketed, to be actually used.

Importing specific types of microflora, like in the cases of kombucha and kefir, allows us to predict and benefit from their actions. Utilizing wild bacteria, however, yields a universe of flavors and health benefits that we can suppose and experience, but to a full extent only imagine. Fermented vegetables in Ecuador will have a different community of probiotics than ones from Alaska, and so a different taste and effect on our health. And so much the better, if the people consuming them are in Ecuador and Alaska. By eating local fermentations of wild bacteria, you'll connect on the deepest level with your community and build immunity to pathogens and allergens that the local bacteria have already overcome. You'll invite the untamed life force of the natural world to your table and body, especially important in the urban jungle where the only wilderness hides on this microscopic level.

Fermenting vegetables is a simple process (from a human point of view) though a very rewarding one, and no special equipment is needed. Just a vessel to hold the vegetables, some salt to keep out unwanted organisms, and a way to keep the veggies down. I started with gallon olive jars, gotten for free from bars, and rocks. Not rocket science. The salt can be either sea salt (preferred) or pickling salt, which is table salt without the added iodine, an anti-microbial agent. Kosher salt can also be used, but as the grains are much bigger and have less surface area for the mass, about 50% is needed.

Any fruit or vegetable can be fermented, but let's start with sauerkraut made from cabbage. Enjoyed all over the world and a welcome addition to many foods you probably already eat; cabbage is inexpensive and already rich in the lacto-bacillus that will team up with your local wild flora. In my opinion, cabbage is by far the world's #1 fermented veggie because its glucosamines (see "what to sprout" in "Kitchen Sink Farming Volume 1: Sprouting") act as a natural pesticide, deterring larger bugs from populating and leaving room for the probiotics to flourish. Others believe that cabbage, being an autumn and early-winter vegetable, was a better candidate for long-term storage by pre-fridge cultures, and the world has developed a taste for it. The reason why sauerkraut and its incarnations in various cultures is so good may be a matter of debate; the fact that it *is* so good is just common knowledge.

Basic Sauerkraut Recipe

You'll need:

One head of cabbage per 1 quart of container, 4 heads for a gallon jar

1 ½ Tbl Sea Salt per head of cabbage

Chop or grate the cabbage. Thick or thin, with the heart or without; whatever you prefer. The light green and dark purple varieties are interchangeable, and can be mixed to make a light pink kraut. Other chopped or grated veggies, fruits, or sprouted seeds can be thrown in now as well; garlic, beets, carrots, greens (mustard and others), apples, seaweeds, or herbs like dill or sprouted celery seed are common options.

Why Salt?

For the biochemistry–minded, salt is added to fermenting veggies and fruits for two reasons. One is to induce osmosis; the fluid inside of the plant material will be sucked out in nature's desire to balance salt content on both sides of the cell wall, and the resulting liquid is wonderfully full of sugars and growth-promoting factors. The other reason is that salt will inhibit the growth of spoilage microorganisms and pathogens. The lacto bacteria that turn fermented fruits and veggies into delicious sauerkraut or pickled tangerines, for examples, are already present on the skin and leaves of all produce.

But again, as humanity, and un-aided nature actually, has been fermenting for longer than the word osmosis existed, it's not necessary to understand the principals behind the process, it's just important to do it. As the old yoga aphorism says: "99% practice, 1% theory".

Toss the cabbage with the salt. Pack it tightly into your container and find something to hold it down like a plate that fits inside your container with a rock on top. The combination of pressure and salt will draw out the liquid; eventually we want everything submerged under the anaerobic protection of salt water.

The easiest, and cleanest method (besides a fermenting crock) is to fill a sprouting or produce bag (see "Resources") with the chopped veggies and weigh it down with a heavy rock that's been sterilized. The best rocks I've found are the smooth round rocks businesses use in their landscaping, about the size of a fist. I'm positive that they'll give you a couple if you ask nicely. To sterilize your rock, scrub it with dish soap and hot water, then put it in a pot of boiling water for 10 minutes, covering the rock completely. You can also put the rock in an oven set to 350° F for 15 minutes. BE VERY CAREFUL as the rock could have air bubbles inside which will heat, expand, and explode. Wrap the rock in a dishtowel, which won't burn until it reaches 450, and will possibly contain an explosion.

Other Methods:

As the veggies are acted upon by the breathing bacteria, bubbles will attach to individual shreds of leaf, which will want to float to the surface of the water. At this point, the guides say to put a plate on top of the cabbage that just fits inside of the container and weigh it down with a rock. I've never been able to find so perfect a match. Even grated

vegetables held down by a well-fitting plate will often find an opening, and like weeds growing up through the crack in a sidewalk will find their way to the surface and out of the safety of the brine. Veggies in a sprouting bag won't have this problem. Another option is to fill a plastic freezer bag with brine (in case it leaks) and use this to hold down the veggies; the benefit (besides being cheap and already in your possession) is a complete seal. The drawback is a messy surface; often a harmless white mold will form where the water meets air. This bloom should be scooped out as soon as it forms to allow the bacteria under the water free access to oxygen, which is why I like to keep the surface of the water free from obstructions. If you let the mold overgrow, it can smell quite bad and cleaning is more difficult. I use my plastic strainer (the same one I use for my kefir) to skim the surface. The plastic makes it easy to squeeze it into the vessel, if the mouth is not as wide as the body. Rinse it upside down with hot water in between scoops. You can also use a very clean cloth for each pass. The plastic bag technique makes cleaning virtually impossible, and if it's in and out of the water as handfuls of kraut are scooped out every once in a while, it'll turn messy fast.

The last option I've tried is a bottle that fits inside the mouth of the fermenting vessel, filled with water, holding everything down. This has the same problems as the plastic bag but to a lesser degree, as it can be easily and cleanly pulled out and replaced after the mold has been cleaned from it and the water. I've found that Voss water bottles fit pretty well into wide mouthed canning jars (which have the same sized mouth in both the quart and half gallon size), but the most perfectly-fitted bottles are Corralejo tequila, with beautiful bubbly, colored glass. Keep out bugs by covering the whole thing with a clean piece of cloth, clean old t-shirt, or a coffee filter is nothing sticks out over the rim, and rubber-band it down. Put the vessel on a plate or shallow bowl, in case of spills or

overflow. Or, if the vessel has a lid, screw it on. The fermentation that's going to happen in this case is anaerobic, so it doesn't need oxygen.

Through osmosis and pressure, the liquid will slowly draw out of the vegetables. Push down on the weight every couple of hours to squeeze out the water, either with a clean hand or kitchen tool; the tamper from a high-speed blender works well. This is the main benefit from using a bottle; very easy to grab it like a dry handle and press down. Be careful not to raise the level of the water so much that it spills out! If after 24-48 hours the vegetables aren't entirely submerged in their own juice, add more brine, 1 cup of fresh water to ¾ tablespoons of salt. Wine can be substituted for the extra brine; it will give the kraut a more delicate taste that some who haven't yet acquired a taste for strong fermented flavors may appreciate.

Cover the whole thing with a towel or t-shirt to prevent bugs from getting in and leave your veggies to ferment. A dark corner of a kitchen counter works well; a cool cupboard is also good. Probiotics like darkness and 60-75° Fahrenheit. The colder the temperature the slower the fermentation process, which can make a mellower flavored kraut. Above 75 or 80° and a new type of bacteria will feel at home, which could be a problem.

Your kraut or other fermented veggies will start to be ready in just a few days, and will continue to mature for months. If you're going to let them go that long, you will want to look for a cool place to let them work, after the initial few days of getting started in the kitchen. I like to start eating my kraut in about a week, and keep dipping in until it's gone. I start a batch of something when I'm nearing the end of the last, so that I always have something working (usually several somethings). Whenever a friend has an over-abundance of a fruit of vegetable, or when I get a great deal at a farmer's market at the end of the day, it gets fermented.

The original reason people started fermenting, a way to store produce for when times were lean, is still a great reason to do it. Delicate greens will last a few days in the fridge, or months in the fermenter. Wherever you live, fruits and vegetables are only available certain times of the year, and are shipped in from across the globe during the others. An expensive process, both to the wallet and the environment. While the health benefits of fermented veggies are many, the environmental benefits may be even greater.

Sterilization

When a home fermenter wants only beneficial organisms in their brew, they need to work with clean tools. This way, they can make sure that no soil-based organisms, for example, are going to be competing with the lacto-bacteria in a vegetable culture, or that the delicate yeasts and bacteria in a young kombucha culture won't have to fight with free-floating mold spores as they establish themselves. Obviously, sterilization is a new process, and judging from the millennia of successful fermentation that happened before its discovery, not a totally necessary one. But it does make the process simpler and more consistent. There are four ways to sterilize your equipment, boiling, baking, chemicals, or UV light. Bacteria can't survive past 250° F (120° C) for any length of time, at least the ones we're generally exposed to, so boiling your jars, bags, rocks, etc., for 10 minutes will do the trick. Tools can also be sterilized in an oven, which takes longer because any cooling water in or on the object must evaporate before the desired temperature can be reached, about 2 hours at 300° F. I also have a UV sterilizer wand that is fast and handy; about a minute per jar does the trick, and it's convenient to use on kitchen sponges, hotel pillows, or other places unwanted bacteria might develop. Simply washing equipment with hot water will almost always be enough, but an ounce of prevention is worth it in the case of weeks or months-long ferments.

Hydrogen peroxide (see "Kitchen Sink Farming Volume 3: Growing"), iodine, colloidal silver, or a citrus-based commercial sanitizer can also be used.

Now that you're an expert in fermenting veggies at home, try these:

Kimchi – cabbage, carrot, ginger, garlic, onion, chili

Cabbage with apple, cranberries (halved), and a bit of shallot

Tangerines with cinnamon, clove, and honey

Cabbage, shredded carrot, onion, radish, and ginger

Carrots, beets, and raisins

Cultural diversity is as important in our guts as it is in our communities!

Fermented veggies and wonderful on their own, on a slice of sprouted bread or dried cracker, or in many recipes but fermented condiments might be the apex of the art. A perfect blend of sweet and sour that enliven any food, the following condiment ideas will hopefully inspire you to include a dollop of a fermented goodness on the side of every meal. Even cereal and desserts will benefit from "Almond Cream Cheese" (see "Kitchen Sink Farming Volume 4: Homegrown Living Recipes - What to Do with Your Sprouts and Krauts").

Try these:

Raisins, garlic chives, cilantro, sprouted anise and cumin, ginger, whey (see Kitchen Sink Farming Volume 3: Fermenting)

Plum and Apple Chutney with carrot, cinnamon, allspice, ginger, and blackberries

Apricot and Rosemary

Green Tomato and Basil

Celery-Pear

Seed Cheese and Yogurt

Fermenting sprouted seeds and nuts into a creamy vegan cheese takes them to the next level in nutrition, digestibility, and epicure. Macadamia nuts can transform into a delicious crumbly feta, and quinoa, hemp and corn can become a full-flavored and velvety cheese spread in just a day or two of fermenting. Using the air-born beneficial organisms that occur naturally in your home, fermented seed cheeses are full of active enzymes, predigested protein, easy-to-assimilate starches, new health-giving nutrients only available through the microbial action, and of course, live probiotic cultures. The "soy cheese" or "cashew cream cheese" in natural food stores or on raw restaurant menus are almost always just blended nuts with dead yeast and flavorings; this is the real deal. Remember – in seeds "raw" means nothing, "alive" means everything.

Simple Seed Cheese

To make cheese, we need to first make probiotic water (recipe above), a simple elixir that develops the existing friendly bacteria on seeds and grains and lures in additional helpers that will go to work for us. Probiotic water is also an easy and effective way to supplant varied bacterial cultures in our digestive systems. It has a light, mild flavor reminiscent of lemon and bread, and can be used instead of plain old water in every juice, soup, or recipe that's not going to be heated past 115° F (as this would kill most of our guests, which is not very polite), or just drunk straight.

The Next Step

Put your sprouted seeds or nuts in a food processor or blender with just enough probiotic water to cover them. Pulse grind them until they're pulverized but not smooth. The right texture is important – the ground mixture needs enough consistency to be homogenous enough to end up a solid mass when the liquid is removed; pureed too thin and it will all drain away. You want a fairly smooth consistency, while still having some texture. If it is over-smooth, throw in some herbs and veggies to thicken it up, and you've got a delicious dip.

Wash the soaking/sprouting jar thoroughly with hot water and return the blended mixture to it. Leave it at least a third empty, as the fermenting cheese will bubble and expand. Re-cover it with the screen, coffee filter, sprout bag or fabric, screw on the ring, and put it in a room temperature place, 65-75° F. If your room is colder than that, the top of your fridge will probably keep it the right temp. If your room is hotter, try a dark closet or clean ground-floor or below-ground corner.

Start checking it at 6 hours. Don't shake, swirl, or otherwise molest your project. The microbes are working hard to make your cheese, and if you disturb them it sets them back. I could image slowing down a fermentation in this way, and I imagine this would make a more sour or pungent finished product. The cheese will be done around 12-24 hours. There will be a thick, light colored mass floating on top of a clearish liquid; the solid is curds, and the liquid is whey.

Now, carefully scoop the cheese out of the jar with a spoon and place it in a sprouting bag or piece of cheesecloth. The top layer of the cheese may be darker from reacting to the oxygen; this is completely fine to eat. If it's dry and crusty you may want to scoop it off first and discard it for aesthetic reasons. Squeeze the rest of the whey out of the cheese into the jar or a separate bowl. Whey will last a really long time in a sealed jar in the fridge, and is great for many recipes, including lacto-ferments and sodas, as well as many household things. The resulting lump of cheese should be dry and have a creamy or crumbly texture, depending on the seed, grain, or nuts used and the original consistency of the mixture. It's ready to be used immediately, can be mixed with flavoring agents like salt, soy sauce, lemon juice, peppers or herbs and spices, and stored for up to a week.

Crumble seed cheese on salads and soups or use it in wraps or as a spread on veggies or crackers – anytime you'd use dairy cheese but still want to feel non-mucousy and deeply nourished. Actually, seed cheese is so high in available protein and so easy to digest that many people have trouble keeping on weight, and body builders alike find that seed cheese is the best source for lean muscles, especially when made from hemp (see Kitchen Sink Farming Volume 1: Sprouting).

As we've discussed, the cheese is highly reactive with air, so put it in a sealed container in the fridge; I don't recommend wrapping the lump of cheese with plastic which may leach harmful chemicals into the food, but the less air there is in the container, the less drying out there will be.

Seed Cheese Recap

You'll need:

A cup of sprouted seeds, nuts, or grains

About 1/3 cup of probiotic water (see pg 64)

Do:

In a blender or food processor, cover the sprouts with the probiotic water. Gently pulse the blades until the mixture is a fairly smooth consistency, while still having some texture.

Clean the sprouting jar and return the mixture to it. Re-cover with a breathable material and place in a temperate spot, 65-75° F.

Your ferment is done when the mixture separates, curds floating on top of whey. Saving the liquid whey, scoop out the curds and squeeze dry in a sprouting bag.

"Advanced" Cheese Making: A 2-Day Degree

While simple seed cheese makes a quick and creamy result, colander cheese will produce a more intensely cheesy concoction, as the flavors develop slowly over the course of a few days, "pre-digesting" and breaking down the complex elements all the while. Still a very straight-forward and easy recipe, colander cheese is the gourmet's choice.

What you'll need:

Sprouted grains and/or nuts and probiotic water, as mentioned above;

A colander with legs, or some sort of strainer and a way to keep it lifted, like crossed chopsticks or rocks (or just go buy a colander with legs, they're like a buck);

A bowl that fits nicely inside the colander;

A heavy weight: a clean rock, jar or bottle filled with water, etc.; and

A plate or shallow bowl to go underneath the colander.

Blend your soaked and/or sprouted seeds or nuts with the probiotic water into a smooth mixture that still has some texture (see simple seed cheese recipe above), and put the resulting half creamy, half chunky, and all wet paste back into a sprout bag, twisting or tying off the opening so nothing comes out. Put it into the colander. The plate or shallow bowl goes underneath to catch the whey, and the bowl goes inside the colander, on top of the bag. The weight goes in the bowl, which presses down on the cheese to squeeze out the whey.

Over the next 2 – 3 days, all of the whey created by the fermentative action of the bacteria will drain out of the cheese. It's a good idea to stir or knead the cheese once a day so it will ferment evenly. After the whey stops dripping into the vessel beneath, the cheese is done and can be scooped out and put into a non-plastic container in the fridge, or formed into logs and rolled in herbs, crushed black pepper, the same type of seed or nut, coarsely ground and dried, or whatever flavoring you choose.

Coconut Cream Cheese

This is a different process that slowly produces an incredible sweet cheese from coconut pudding. I discovered this cheese by accident, when some pudding was starting to go south after a week or so, and I went out of town, resolving to throw it away when I got back about a week later. When I returned home I found a jar full of coconut puree in my refrigerator with a fuzzy growth on top, varying in color from white to dark brown. As I started scooping the stuff into the garbage disposal, I fortuitously caught a whiff of it as it went by. It smelled sweet and delicious, and I decided to try it. I scraped all the fuzz off the top and tasted a small spoonful. It was amazing, and as much as I wanted more, I waited to see how I felt. The next day I felt great, so I ate a bunch. Still fine, so now coconut cheese is a staple in my repertoire.

Make coconut pudding by blending young coconut meat with its water (see "Kitchen Sink Farming Volume 4: Homegrown Living Recipes – What to Do with Your Sprouts and Krauts"). A fairly thick consistency works best, as it gives the microbes something to adhere to. Scoop it into a jar and cover it with a screen, cheesecloth, sprout bag, or coffee filter so that your local flora will appear. If you're doing this in a sterile environment like outer space and don't have access to helpful organisms, or as an experiment, you can also use *koji*, a mold used to make sake and amasake, fermented rice beverages from Japan, available online or from some home brewing stores.

Leave the pudding on a counter for 12-24 hours, cover the jar with a lid, and put in the fridge. You'll start to see growth in about 2 weeks, and the flavor will continue to develop as the microorganisms turn the complex carbohydrates into sugars, and in turn digests the sugars. When you're ready to use it, scrape the top layer off, cleaning off the spoon or spatula between scrapings. Still not as gross as bleu cheese or moldy green-veined ones.

The coconut cream cheese is ready to be used in desserts or to sweeten up and add a hint of champagne sparkle to spreads for fruits or vegetables. It's really so delicious that it can be served plain in a digestion-boosting scoop, as a side for anything from appetizer to dessert. It's also amazing blended with fresh orange juice, which turns into a tropical creamsicle, and (fortunately or unfortunately) covers up the fermented flavor.

Vinegar

For thousands of years, vinegar held a prime place on the healer's shelves for its many health benefits, and at some point found its way into the chef's tool kit as well. Its low pH (high acidity) stimulated digestion by giving a boost to the stomach acids, and it's been used over the centuries to treat everything from skin conditions like warts and eczema to internal issues like arthritis, infections, headaches, high cholesterol, and ulcers. Apple cider vinegar is a popular and effective elixir, especially as a weight loss aid because of its bowel stimulating and appetite suppressing qualities. It's been studied less, but I find kombucha vinegar equal to apple cider in benefits and taste. Many pet owners have noticed increased energy and shinier coats in their dogs, cats, horses, birds, and rodents when apple cider vinegar is added to their pet food, and the ancient Samurai, sadly unmentioned in the rest of this book, believed a daily shot of vinegar would increase their vitality and power in battle (tamago-su or egg vinegar, was made by dissolving a whole raw egg in rice vinegar for a week).

Vinegar is any acidic, or low pH, liquid that contains acetic acid, and along with lemons is the only very acid food. For this reason, it's irreplaceable for adding zip to many dishes, soups, sauces, and of course vinaigrettes. And luckily, it's so easy to make that juice and wine makers have to take precautions to make sure their products *don't* turn into it. It could be said that the sugars in many liquid foods will turn into acetic acid by accident, but consistently making a nice, mellow vinegar with just the right amount of bite takes just a little bit of knowledge.

Any liquid with some sugar (or carbohydrates, aka starch, which is sugar molecules bound in groups, so another step is required to make the sugars available) can become vinegar, from all kinds of fruit and vegetable juices (common ones are apple and grape), grains like wheat or rice, or sweeteners like honey, molasses, agave, or sugarcane. Even vinegars made from roots, bark, and wood were once very popular. The two-step process of turning the sugar into alcohol, and the alcohol into acetic acid yields the most consistent outcome (like grape juice into wine into red wine vinegar), but just combining an active vinegar starter with any of the above liquids and letting them brew will usually give fine results.

We'll start with the more complicated version so you'll understand the process, maybe keeping it in the back of your mind until you'd like to try your hand at an exceptional vinegar for a special occasion. Also, this process doesn't need a starter culture to get going; it makes the most of the natural yeasts and bacteria that are present in the air. The super-easy classic Kitchen-Sink Farmer follows.

First, you'll need a sweet liquid: a sweetener like honey, molasses, maple syrup or sugar and water, or fruit or vegetable juice. Apple juice has a good balance of sugars and acids that make it an ideal choice for a first vinegar. Put the liquid in a clean bottle or jug, filling it all the way up to the top. Next, you'll need an airlock which lets carbon dioxide out but doesn't let oxygen in. These are available from homebrew stores, and are a curved tube with water inside. The water lets the CO2 bubble away, but air (particularly oxygen) can't pass through in the other direction. You can also make your own airlock, of course, by drilling a hole in a rubber stopper, a wine bottle cork, a cornhusk, or piece of soft wood carved to fit the bottleneck. Put a piece of flexible plastic tubing (available from hardware, medical supply or aquarium stores) into the hole and put the other end into a glass of water. Air can get out but not in. DIY airlock - check!

As the fermentation begins, you'll notice bubbling in the water. This, as mentioned, is CO2, a waste product being emitted by the microorganisms. The other waste product is alcohol, and when the bubbling stops (2-4 weeks, depending on how much sugar is in your original liquid) you have made alcohol. Hard cider if you've used apple juice, mead if you've used honey water, etc. You have probably already realized, but your newfound tools and knowledge of yeast fermentation can be applied to all kinds of homemade wines. Wine or champagne can also be used to make vinegar by simply starting with the next step.

The next phase is to turn the alcohol into acetic acid, the classic flavor that's consistent throughout all vinegars.

This process uses a new set of microorganisms that thrive in the presence of oxygen, or aerobically. The more oxygen these organisms can use, the faster the fermentation will happen, so you'll want to maximize the surface area of the brew. Pour the liquid into a wide-mouth jar or bucket, or divide it into a few bottles. Cover the opening with a light cloth or coffee filter secured by a rubber band and leave it for as long as you like. If you have some vinegar starter, or "mother" it can be added to speed up the process. It will, after a couple of weeks, continue to get stronger and more acidic, and will quickly surpass the potency of store-bought vinegars. It can even be looked at as a "vinegar concentrate", with water or juice added to achieve the desired zip. Bottle and cap it when it's reached the strength you like, and because it won't have access to oxygen it won't get any stronger but will continue to deepen in flavor as its bottle-aged. After you're adept at this process, you may like to flavor your vinegar between steps 2 and 3, "acetic acid fermentation" and bottling, by putting herbs, fruit, sprouted grains, chilies, horseradish, onions, garlic, flowers, or other flavorings in the vinegar for a day to a week. These will add another layer of sophistication and potentially a lovely color to your homemade brew. The finished product can be so beautiful that you're tempted to put it in clear glass and display it, but remember that sunlight can break down living vinegar.

The yeast and acetic acid fermentation can also be done at the same time, but this process is just a little more fickle. If you're a gamblin' man (or lady), you can just put juice in a wide-mouthed jar, cover it with an air-permeable light cloth, and leave it for a few weeks, letting the different stages of microbia come and go. If the surface gets covered by a very fuzzy layer that breaks up when you swirl it, this is a somewhat volatile wild yeast and it's best to abandon the project. If a SCOBY forms in the juice (symbiotic colony or bacteria and yeast, like a rubbery white pancake) you've created a thriving metropolis of beneficial organisms, and you'll soon have delicious vinegar. A bit of this living condiment can be saved and added to the next brew as a starter. If possible, I recommend adding an unpasteurized, unfiltered vinegar at the outset of a vinegar brew to solidify the bacteria's foothold in its new colony. Unpasteurized apple cider vinegar is the most commonly available in stores, with "Bragg Organic Raw Apple Cider Vinegar" being the most widely available. Whether you used a store-bought or homemade starter, the easiest way to stay in vinegar is to do a continuous fermentation: when you take some vinegar out of your jar, add some new juice, as mentioned in the sections on kombucha and kefir. You will be missing the mellowing effect of bottling with this method, but once you've established your culture, continuous fermentation makes it a snap to keep it going forever.

Vinegar can also be made with kitchen scraps and peels, already full of beneficial bacteria because of their exposure to the air while growing. If you've washed your fruit and veggies in hydrogen peroxide (see "Kitchen Sink Farming Volume 3: Growing") you're guaranteed the lack of uncooperative anaerobic bacteria (oxygen-hating) while maintaining the aerobic ones (oxygen-loving). Put the peels and scraps in a wide mouthed jar and cover with filtered water and a light cloth or coffee filter. Continue to throw in kitchen scraps now and then to give the bacteria new sugars to feed off of. Start tasting the brew after a few weeks (dip a straw into the liquid then cover the end with your finger. You'll be able to lift the full straw out without losing any liquid, uncovering it when the bottom end is in your mouth. This testing method is called "thieving" in wine-making.) In 4-6 weeks it should be done. Apple cores and peels work especially well for this method, as well as peaches, pears, apricots, crushed grapes, and berries. If you don't like the taste of your kitchen-scrap vinegar, it's also an excellent plant nutrient.

Vinegar Flies

Wherever there's vinegar brewing, these pesky little friends (sometimes called fruit flies) show up. They love fermentation almost as much as I do, which is why they're often found around overripe bananas and oranges, or getting funky on an old batch of collard greens. I used to try to catch them in my fist and put them outside, until I learned that these are the critters most commonly used in labs to study genetics because of their short life cycle and hardiness. Then I thought: if I remove all the slow ones, leaving just the fast ones to reproduce, I'm inadvertently breeding a super-strain of ninja gnats. I've found that the best way to deal with them without direct violence is to put some vinegar in a glass or bowl and cover it with plastic wrap. Then poke a bunch of holes in the top with a fork (a piece of paper rolled into an downward-pointing cone with a small hole in the tip, above the level of the liquid, also works). The flies can get in but they can't get out. Kind of mean, but they are vinegar flies, after all, so I bet they die happy.

Super-Easy Apple Cider Vinegar

Get a bottle of raw apple cider vinegar

> Add it to a bottle of apple juice (no preservatives)
>
> Cover with a cloth and let ferment.
>
> Easy!

To make **wild fermented apple cider vinegar** and enjoy all the immunity-boosting and evolutionary benefits of aligning with your local flora, juice apples, which have probiotics and yeasts on their peels. You may also buy apple juice (with no preservatives, refrigerated means fresh). Wash and cut up an apple and put it in a bowl or wide-mouth jar, and fill with apple juice. Cover with a clean cloth and let it sit for a week or more, swirling the liquid a couple of times a day to inhibit mold (if a layer of white mold does grow on the surface, it can be scooped off). Continue to ferment until it gets the acidity you like, then cover and stick in the fridge. Will stay "good" forever.

Special Vinegars

White wine vinegar is made by pouring double the amount of water over mashed raisins and leaving it for about 2 months. Strain the pulp out and use it again and again. Make raspberry vinegar by using fresh raspberries. Everyday for three days, add the same amount of fresh berries and enough water to cover. On day four, strain the liquid out and add one pound of sugar or honey, stirring until dissolved. Cover with a light cloth or coffee filter until it turns to vinegar - this takes about three months.

Make a lovely flower vinegar by dissolving (preferably raw) honey in twice the amount of warm pure water, less than 110° F, so as not to kill the living organisms. Of course, any natural sweetener will do; raw honey isn't necessary for the process but it's just so much better for you and since it's made from pollen, goes wonderfully with the floral taste of this brew. Add several handfuls of edible flowers like marigold, clover, dandelions, nasturtium, citrus blossoms, jasmine, or herb flowers or leaves. Cover with a coffee filter or cloth and stir or swirl every day until it's done, usually 10 to 20 days. Strain the liquid and bottle it, though you may want to leave a particularly beautiful stem in the bottle, especially if the vinegar is a gift.

If you're curious about the actual acidity of your vinegar, which is a great way to determine if it's ready, there are three methods of finding out. One is a pH test kit, where a litmus paper will change color and tell you the acidity. There's also titration, a process using baking soda that determines the strength of the acid in the solution by finding out the smallest amount that's required to react with the baking soda (remember vinegar or lemon juice and baking soda volcanoes from middle school?). Instructions are available online and the benefit is that you only need household items: jars, water, baking soda, and a colored liquid of some kind. The other method is a laboratory pH tester, which starts at about $20, and I find extremely handy in all sorts of projects. I use my pH tester to determine when my brews are done, from kombucha to kefir to kraut, and I highly recommend picking one up. The pH tester won't tell you how much of *which kind* of acid is present, but that you can easily figure out by taste if you're interested.

Mead and Ginger Beer

Mead, or honey wine, is the simplest process described in this book, and by far the easiest thing you'll ever do that results in something to sip or chew (and that includes microwaving a tv dinner).   And though it's so easy to do, perhaps *because* of it, brewing your own mead, like enjoying a sunset or howling at the moon, is participating in the most original amusement of our species.   Some anthropologists believe that mead altered the course of humanity more than any other factor.

Raw honey is full of both probiotic bacteria and natural antibiotics that protect it from invasion by other microbial species. In fact, several-thousand years old honey was found in Egyptian tombs, quite fresh.   But when wild honey mixes with water by nature or human design, it dilutes honey's natural protections so that wild yeasts and bacteria are able to get in to the candy store and enjoy the sweet nectar, converting it in their special way into a bubblingly living ferment. In just a few days to a few weeks,

"I in my grandeur have surpassed the heavens and all this spacious earth.

Have I not drunk of Soma juice?

…O Soma flowing on thy way, win thou and conquer high renown; And make us better than we are.

Win thou the light, win heavenly light, and, Soma, all felicities; And make us better than we are.

…When purified within the jars, Soma,… golden-hued… flow on to us and make us rich. Drive all our enemies away.

… Send down the rain from heaven, a stream of opulence from earth."

Soma Pavamana, HYMN IV.

the honey-water will be mead, its sugars having been converted to alcohol and CO_2 by the action of the microorganisms.

The theory is that a caveperson happened upon a bubbling, golden liquid in the crook of a tree: honey that had been rained on, and was now being transformed by invisible forces. The caveperson carefully tried it, liked it, tried some more. Maybe the caveperson called some cave friends over and a cave party ensued, complete with, as is the case with many neophytic drinkers, much rowdiness, finding formerly uninteresting things fascinating, and animated declarations of love. The intoxicating elixir was seen as a mysterious gift from the gods. Songs were sung, offerings made. Actually, it's interesting to note that the *Vedas*, the large body of poems from ancient India (called apauruṣeya or "not of human agency") that kicked off the Hindu religion and influenced all the other ones, were unabashedly written under the influence of a mysterious drug called "soma", literally "juice" or "nectar" in Sanskrit, which historians believe was either mead or the juice of the ephedra plant, pounded out of the stalks, filtered, fermented and mixed with milk.

By some accounts, it was not the cultivation of crops or livestock, but the desire for the altered state that fermentation provides that inspired primitive nomadic man to decide to stay put. Mead, which predates the cultivation of fire, influenced our hunter-gatherer ancestors to convert from a wandering lifestyle to a sedentary one, a way of life that had been working for at least 2 million years. It was this shift that cultural theorist Claude Levi-Strauss says marks the transition from nature to culture in prehistoric man. Describing a hollow tree he writes, "…which, as a receptacle for honey, is part of nature if the honey is fresh and enclosed within it, and part of culture if the honey, instead of being in a naturally hollow tree, has been put to ferment in an artificially hollowed-out trunk" (*From Honey to Ashes*, 1973).

Mead was also my first attempt at fermentation, as a teenaged way to get an alcoholic buzz and, I like to think, the buzz that a curious soul gets from cultivating mysterious forces. A friend of the family described to me the process in a few sentences, my curiosity was peeked, and I gathered my materials: a gallon water jug and a plastic bear container of honey that had been collecting dust and crystallizing in our kitchen pantry for as long as I could remember. The honey went into the jug which was then filled with water, and I put it under my bed, checking it every day when I got home from school. I noticed it start to bubble after a few days, and though I didn't understand why (wild yeasts, which had floated on the air towards the sweet vapors like the steam from a cartoon pie, were releasing carbon dioxide), I knew that *something* was happening, much like my ancient ancestors probably did. I watched the bubbling decrease over the course of a couple of weeks, both hesitant and fascinated. When I finally worked up the nerve to take a sip, I was surprised to find that it wasn't sweet at all, for the same reason that it had stopped bubbling: the yeasts had eaten all the sugars. I wasn't ready for the exotic taste exposed by the removal of the sugar, nor the layer of bugs that had sunk to the bottom of the jug. I tossed the mixture (probably a good thing, or I'd still have the toxic PCBs in my fat cells that had been leached out of the soft plastic) and didn't come back to the memory for about ten years, when I had learned enough to use a glass jug and cover the mouth. Now it's ten years after that and I'm playing with herb and fruit flavorings, homemade airlocks, and different kinds of honey. And the evolution of our species continues.

Mead recipe not in story form:

Ingredients:

A 1 gallon glass juice jug or jar, or a 5 gallon glass water jug (harder to find, a hard plastic one will also work, but don't let the ferment get too acidic or it will begin to leach the plastic)

3 cups or 750 mL of honey, preferably raw

A breathable piece of cloth, coffee filter, or sprouting bag

A rubber band and the jug's lid (you can also cover the opening with your palm during shaking, if you don't have the lid)

Directions:

Put the honey in the jug, fill with water, cap it. Shake it vigorously until the honey is dissolved. Remove the lid and secure the breathable material over the opening with the rubber band.

Put it in a warm place, out of the sun, and swirl it a couple of times a day to keep it mixed and aerated. The more oxygen and honey the yeasts can get at, the faster the fermentation. You can also stir it with a clean, long spoon.

In a few days you'll notice gentle bubbling; it will slow down and eventually stop over the course of 2 or 3 weeks. The brew will become less sweet the longer it ferments. Start tasting it after 2 weeks, and you'll notice it becoming drier, higher in alcohol, and more viscous. There's no rule about when it's best enjoyed, and it's nice to have a little bit of simple, plain mead every few days and experience the arc of its life cycle.

Flavoring Your Mead

Other ingredients can be added at various points in the process; adding fresh foods to mead or vinegar was once necessary to preserve them; it's likely that appreciation for the new flavors came second. It's easiest to add berries, herbs, fruits, roses, etc., along with the water at the beginning of the brewing process, though much of the flavor will go out of them as their sugars are used as a food source by the yeasts along with the honey. Adding flavoring agents at or towards the end will generally yield a more flavorful brew, though you may want to play with partially or fully fermenting extra ingredients for added flavor, kick, and medicinal benefits. Be careful though, because many delicious herbal and medicinal flavorings are actually anti-microbial, and will prevent the fermentation process altogether. Cloves, eucalyptus, chilis, garlic, lemon, burdock, marigold, and grapefruit seed are anti-microbial, so add them only after the initial fermentation.

When fruit is being used as an ingredient, it has the habit of floating on top of the mead, creating what is called a "cap". This can cause a couple of issues with the fermentation, the most crucial of which is the potential for contamination. When the cap sits for an extended period of time on top of the mead, it can begin to dry out, creating a crust on which mold can grow. This mold will then contaminate the mead, creating off flavors and potential health risks. The cap can also restrict the bubbling off of the carbon dioxide, which will build up in the mead and slow down the fermentation. To prevent the cap from drying out and to aid in the release of the CO_2, the cap needs to be punched down a couple of times a day. This requires nothing more than to gently stir the fruit back down into the mead using a clean spoon.

Adding pureed ingredients anytime before the very end will make them ferment too quickly, the bacteriological equivalent of putting a bunch of toddlers in a pool filled with cotton candy. Freezing pieces of fruits or whole berries will burst their cell walls and make the juices more available to the fermentation, while decelerating the process by giving their cellular innards a little privacy. Traditional flavors include apple and cinnamon, the lemon herbs (-grass, -thyme, -basil, -balm, and -verbena), and mulling spices. I've tried lemon/ginger, raspberry/tangerine/goat milk kefir (citrus is best sliced into disks, peel on), clove/cinnamon, and cacao/mint, and like them all. Some people even throw in multi-vitamins, why the heck not? The following is a recipe from Edward Spencer's "The Flowing Bowl", 1903:

"Take of spring water what quantity you please, and make it more than blood-warm, and dissolve honey in it til 'tis strong enough to bear an egg, the breadth of a shilling; then boil it gently near an hour, taking off the scum as it rises; then put to about nine or ten gallons seven or eight large blades of mace, three nutmegs quartered, twenty cloves, three or four sticks of cinnamon, two or three roots of ginger, and a quarter of an ounce of Jamaica pepper; put these spices into the kettle to the honey and water, a whole lemon, with a sprig of sweet-briar and a sprig of rosemary; tie the briar and rosemary together, and when they have boiled a little while take them out and throw them away; but let your liquor stand on the spice in a clean earthen pot till the next day; then strain it into a vessel that is fit for it; put the spice in a bag, and hang it in the vessel, stop it, and at three months draw it into bottles. Be sure that 'tis fine when 'tis bottled; after 'tis bottled six weeks 'tis fit to drink."

"Wine is constant proof that God loves us and loves to see us happy. -Benjamin Franklin

Works for me. Note – most mead recipes recommend boiling honey, which kills all the bacteria and yeasts already present. This allows for an easier foothold for the wild yeasts that come in to ferment the mead. This may be true but I dislike removing any benefits, and as mentioned in the section about raw honey (see "Kitchen Sink Farming Volume 4: Homegrown Living Recipes – What to Do with Your Sprouts and Krauts") heating honey can release toxin compounds the bees picked up from the flowers they visited. I prefer honey raw, unadulterated and alive.

Alcohol

The alcohol content of your mead is determined by a couple of different things. First, the kinds of yeasts that are in your brew have different tolerances to alcohol, which is their waste product (along with CO_2), and poisonous to them. Once the level of alcohol goes higher than their ability to live in it, they will die and their contribution to the ferment will end. These tolerances are well-documented in commercial yeast, but in wild fermentations every batch can be excitingly unpredictable.

The second factor is how much honey is in the brew. A starting ratio of more water to less honey will give the yeasts less food to convert to alcohol, and therefore lower alcohol in the finished product. More honey will yield the opposite result. More honey can also be added a few times during the fermentation, which will make the mead both sweeter and higher in alcohol. It's important to note that the higher the alcohol content, the less susceptible your mead will be to unwanted secondary fermentation, that is, new wild microorganisms coming into your mature brew and producing less-than-desirable flavors.

Once the fermentation has slowed, the bubbles being few, you can enjoy your mead right away or bottle it, or just remove the permeable top from the mouth of the container and screw on a lid, another reason I use canning jars for everything. Since the CO_2 has nowhere to go, it will build pressure and create a slightly sparkling beverage. It can also be strained to remove the cloudy sediment and yeasty flavor common in high-end champagne but that some people don't love.

"It has been my experience that folks who have no vices have very few virtues." - Abraham Lincoln

Other flavors can be added at this time, or more honey or other sweetener to start an anaerobic secondary fermentation. Fruit juice fills both categories.

The exact alcohol content can be measured with a handy tool called a hydrometer, which measures the specific gravity, or thickness, of a liquid. Since alcohol is thicker and stickier than water, it's as easy as measuring before and after.

I'm not going to mention the numerous negative effects of alcohol here, but for our purposes it's worth noting that it can kill the probiotics you've so carefully cultivated in the digestive system. It can also adversely affect every system in the body. But of all libations, home-brewed mead might have the least detriment, and its benefits might possibly tip the scales.

I highly recommend the sections on mead and yeast in "Sacred and Herbal Healing Beers: The Secrets of Ancient Fermentation" by Stephen Harrod Buhner.

Ginger Beer

Ginger beer is a refreshing sparkling soda made with the help of wild yeasts. As far as I've seen, even the best bottled ginger ales sold today use cultivated yeasts and cream of tartar, and so lack the olde-timey flavor that makes authentic, wild ginger beer so special. Once again, the best foods and drinks are only available to the DIY-er and their friends, and for a fraction of the price of the counterfeit.

The first batch of ginger brew requires a "starter" (called a "bug" in Jamaica) which can then be stored for subsequent batches. A starter is a recipe of some sugar and ginger in water that lures the right kind of wild yeasts in. It's handy to have a grater or zester for the ginger (about $10), though it can also be finely chopped or grated with a very clean wood rasp, if you're the type that uses woodworking tools in everyday life. You'll also need some glass bottles that seal, like ones with screw-on lids or bail-wire tops, like old Grolsch beer bottles. The water you use is important; it must be totally free of chlorine so that the yeasts can live and thrive, so if you don't have access to filtered water then get some from the tap and leave it out for 24 hours to let the chlorine evaporate away. A much easier but less traditional and crisp ginger brew can be found in "Kitchen Sink Farming Volume 4: Homegrown Living Recipes – What to Do with Your Sprouts and Krauts".

A slightly more advanced version – worth trying if you're sensitive to sugar is using a combination of raw sugar (also called "turbinado") to feed the yeast, and palm sugar to sweeten the soda; microscopic organisms prefer the simplest form of sugar, which shocks our more complex system.

Ginger Beer Recipe (makes a gallon):

Ingredients

Ginger, skin and all

2 Cups raw sugar (or ½ Cup raw and 1 ½ Cups palm)

2 Lemons

1 Cup Warm Water

Cheesecloth or similar

A small bowl

Bottles

For the "Bug":

Combine 1 cup of pure water, 1 teaspoon grated ginger, and 1 teaspoon raw sugar in a small bowl. Put in a warm place with access to fresh air, like a window sill, and cover with something that will keeps bugs out and let yeasts in, like cheesecloth. Feed the bug every other day by adding another teaspoon each of ginger and sugar and stir, until the liquid starts to bubble, should be between 4 and 8 days. It's most efficient to grate 6 tablespoons of ginger all at once on day one and keep it in the fridge.

The brew can be made anytime the bug is active – keep feeding it until you use it. If you plan on multiple batches, save a few teaspoons of the living starter for future batches in the fridge, where it will stay viable for a couple of weeks.

For the Ginger Brew:

In a pot, combine 2 quarts of water, 2-4 teaspoons grated ginger (depending on how strong you want the ginger flavor) and 1-1 ½ cup sugar (I prefer palm sugar at this point but more raw sugar is fine). Boil the mixture for 15 minutes, then let it cool for about an hour. If you're in a rush, you can use less water then add ice to make up the difference. Make sure the sugar water cools down to less than 110° F, so as not to kill your carefully cultivated bug. It should be a comfortable temperature to your finger. Add the juice of the lemons, a few tablespoons of the strained ginger bug and stir.

Pour the soon-to-be soda into bottles, seal, and leave them to ferment in a warm dark place for 2 weeks or more. There's very little chance of an explosion, but as you're probably using used bottles it's not a bad idea to store them somewhere with detonation in mind, like an unused shower stall or a plastic tote container. Start testing the brew in about a week; the longer it ferments the less sugar and more carbonation it'll have, as the yeasts eat the sugar and produce CO_2. Refrigerate when done to "cold stabilize" the fermentation, and make sure it's cold when opened to avoid a frothy mess.

Fermented Bread

Picture cakey, soft slices of living bread with a hint of sour, slathered with savory vegetable tapenade, rich nut butter, light and velvety clarified butter, or creamy avocado sprinkled with sea salt. As easy as grinding up some sprouted grains and spreading them onto dehydrator trays, the next day pulling off warm, spongy pieces and eating them straight away. Or, painting a thinner layer on the sheet to get crispy crackers. As with everything else in this book, enzyme and nutrient-rich sprouted grain loaves require little time and even less effort, and as we'll see in a moment, the very forces at work might be so misunderstood that they're attributed to gods or angels (though it may be me that doesn't understand). Though we'll cover the history, techniques, and benefits as thoroughly as I know how, this delicious nourishment is mostly the result of experimentation by fairly primitive people. I encourage you to prepare food with as much curiosity and abandon.

Grinding sprouted grains and baking them in the sun is commonly credited to the Essenes, a religious sect that lived near the Dead Sea from 200 BC to 100 AD, though I'm certain that these nutritious living loaves have been around for much longer. Whether or not you stick to raw foods, it might be an unusual experience to eat a couple of slices of moist and flavorful bread and feel light and vibrant afterwards. Sprouting the grain, as discussed in previous chapters, unlocks its full spectrum of nutrition and low temperature baking keeps its living enzymes intact, allowing for complete and effortless digestion and assimilation of all that goodness. We know that enzymes, the chemical components of food that account for its freshness and life begin to degrade at 110° F. However, the same characteristic that allows seeds to go dormant, retaining their potential vitality when sitting for years in the hot sun, can be used for culinary benefit as well.

We first sprout the seeds and grains we'll be using for our breads. Then we slowly turn up the heat, putting the already activated seed *back* into hibernation, allowing for higher-temperature baking that's safe for enzymes. It works like this: if living foods are heated just under 110° F for a half day or so, the enzymes are triggered to go into a dormant state, protecting themselves and their "host" seeds from harm, seeds which we've already made as nutritious and digestible as possible. The heat can be gradually turned up to about 160° F, and the enzymes will stay biologically active. It's a fun experiment: sprout some seeds (I've tried sunflowers, quinoa, and wheat) and separate them into two piles. Put one pile in the dehydrator at 108, or the oven on the "warm" setting, with the door slightly open, and carefully monitor the temperature. After 12 hours, turn up the heat to 150 and put the other group of sprouts in, remembering which group is which. After another day or so, take them out and re-soak them separately for a few hours, then start sprouting them again. You'll notice that the sprouts that were given a low-temp chance to go dormant will continue to sprout, while the other group has passed over to the other side. The group that does sprout will probably do so in a somewhat sluggish and stunted fashion; this can be fixed by slowly turning up the temperature more slowly. It could be quite important to know at what temperature each seed goes dormant and how high its enzymes can survive – please send me the results of your experiments at jp@KitchenSinkFarming.com (and why not subscribe to the blog while you're at it?) and I'll compile a chart so we can know (before we eat them and feel the effects) how to maintain the life-force of our breads. This info might have benefits for storing and distributing high-quality foods in emergency situations as well.

From the Essene Gospels:

"Let the angels of God prepare your bread. Moisten your wheat, that the angels of water may enter it. Then set it in the air, that the angel of air may embrace it. And leave it from morning to evening beneath the sun, that the angel of sunshine may descend upon it. And the blessings of the three angels will soon make the germ of life to sprout in your wheat. Then crush your grain, and make thin wafers, as did your forefathers when they departed out of Egypt, the house of bondage. Put them back again beneath the sun from its appearing, and when it is risen to its highest in the heavens, turn them over on the other side that they may be embraced there also by the angel of sunshine, and leave them there until the sun sets. For the angels of water, and air and of sunshine fed and ripened the wheat in the field, and they likewise must prepare also your bread. And the same sun which, with the fire of life, made the wheat to grow and ripen, must cook your bread with the same fire. For the fire of the sun gives life to the wheat, to the bread, and to the body. But the fire of death kills the wheat, the bread, and the body. And the living angels of the living God serve only living men. For God is the God of the living, and not the God of the dead."

Pretty much the same as what we're saying here, but descriptive in their own way. I wonder why those ancient cookbook writers weren't more specific about what to put the loaf on, how to keep animals away, etc. Maybe it was common knowledge at the time, and in 2000 years people reading this are going to wonder why I didn't explain how to open the refrigerator door. The things we think.

My basic recipe for modern Essene bread calls for 2 cups unsprouted wheat, ¾ cups raisins, and a pinch of sea salt. The wheat is sprouted a little until the root starts to protrude (see "Kitchen Sink Farming Volume 1: Sprouting"), coarsely ground in a food processor or high-speed blender with the raisins, hand-shaped into a loaf, and baked at a low temperature. I find that wheat, with its high gluten content, makes a hearty and dense loaf which some people prefer, but low-temperature air has trouble penetrating to the center. This can be fixed, as in the passage above, by making "thin wafers". I prefer a loafy loaf of bread, with a crisp outer crust and a chewy, slightly moister center, so I go easy on the wheat, instead substituting sprouted grains like quinoa, millet, and amaranth, which have a light texture that allows for low-temperature baking, and a mild nutty flavor that's great in bread.

Naturally Yeasted

The *"it is risen to its highest in the heavens"* part can only refer to fermentation by wild yeast, and one of the best flavorings you can add (or more accurately, "let come in") to your bread. Sprouted breads don't have to be fermented to be nutritious and delicious, but the natural addition of beneficial bacteria will add a layer of health and a natural sourdough flavor so heavenly that you may never want to go a day without it.

If you're going the more traditional route of dehydrator or oven, the exposed fermentation can be duplicated or assisted by first making probiotic water out of the grains and seeds for a few days before grinding them. Bacteria and yeast will cling to the seeds, and they'll be blended into dough that's already biologically active. Obviously, it's better to get into the habit of making each thing for its own benefit and using the leftover "waste" for another project, as opposed to carrying out the several-step process of sprouting grains, then using them to make probiotic water, then making bread out of them, with bread being the purpose of the whole process. Each step has its benefits, and if you have some recently finished grains from probiotic water continuing to gently ferment in the fridge when you run out of bread, you'll be that much more supported by the whole Kitchen Sink Farming process. I prefer using pre-fermented grains than naturally-yeasted bread dough – I'd rather not cruelly tempt those beaks and talons. If I was a bird and found a luminous paste of freshly ground sprouted organic grains and raisins, warmed by the sun, lying out on some dude's balcony, I'd work pretty hard to get at it. If and when we have to find a way to feed ourselves without gas or electricity (or camping, or a fun challenge), I suppose a clear plastic box or large glass vase would do, turned on its side so that the sun can shine through the top and the opening securely covered with a cloth would be a simple solution. A glass-block wall with broken sides could be an effective cookie machine, maybe the easy-bake oven of the future. A birdcage with a shelf inside… Lots of choices abound for enterprising apartment farmers.

See the "Bread, Crusts and Crackers" Section in "Kitchen Sink Farming Volume 4: Homegrown Living Recipes – What to Do with Your Sprouts and Krauts"

Cultivated Flora

As opposed to wild cultures as discussed above, cultivated floras are in their own section because, though they're fermented foods like the rest of this chapter, Kombucha, jun, apple cider vinegar, and kefir are the names given to distinct cultures, colonies of specific bacteria and yeasts that are often thousands of years old, and require a little more initial effort than putting out a bowl of candy and a welcome mat like the rest of our ferments. You'll first have to get a bit of this culture, then give it the opportunity to thrive. This will usually be the traditional method, but there are countless ways to use the culture to ferment other things, like in the case of "coffee-boocha", or kefir-fermented apple butter.

In this section, you'll learn how to find the culture cheaply or freely from locally store-bought products or from folks willing to give the stuff away. The following sections will go over these cultures' many health benefits, safe and simple techniques for home-brewing, ways to procure the culture for cheap or free, and other, secondary products you can make at home with the cultures, like cheese and yogurt in the case of kefir, and vinegar, beer, and champagne ('booch hooch) for the kombucha.

Kombucha

Enjoyed for at least 2,000 years in Asia and Russia, kombucha is rapidly growing in popularity in the rest of the world, where it's sold in natural foods stores for $3-$4 a bottle, though it's really easy to make at home. Many people drink it every day for increased energy, nutrition, immune system and liver function, better digestion, and a plethora of other benefits. Its fermentation is caused by colonies of bacteria and yeasts, all working together and getting along in a way that'd make Rodney King proud, that modern science doesn't fully understand. Though the active organisms are microscopic, the evidence of their cooperation can be easily seen with your own eyes in a quite dramatic way.

The microorganisms in question build a Mother of Kombucha, or "SCOBY", an acronym that stands for "Symbiotic Colony Of Bacteria and Yeasts". More accurately called a "zoogleal mat", this structure resembles a rubbery pancake and isn't the actual culture, but a polysaccharide matrix the organisms build to support themselves, and a really cool indication that something's happening. Even cooler – this germ home will reproduce itself in a week or two so you can start another batch, more quickly ferment in the container you're using, or trade it to someone for something else. The very definition of sustainable all started from a few ounces of a store-bought drink.

To get your very own SCOBY, you'll need to do one of two things. Find someone willing to give or send one to you (try the craig's list barter section or the worldwide kombucha exchange at www.kombu.de). The SCOBY is rich in the organisms that will be brewing your tea, but all that's needed are the organisms, the SCOBY is just a hangout they've built. The easiest method of getting the kombucha creatures is from a bottle of unflavored, unpasteurized kombucha tea, available at most natural food stores, and when conditions are right they'll build a SCOBY on their own. When you buy a bottle of the drink, you're also buying the culture or "seed" which, just like an avocado pit, banana peel, or apple seed, can feed hundreds by cultivating what to most people is something between litter and compost. Be aware that many kombucha companies use an engineered culture designed to be more consistent in terms of fermentation and low alcohol content, but will die off after a couple of brews.

Kombucha Tea Recipe

What you'll need:

5-6 bags of caffeine tea or 10-12 grams of loose tea in a tea ball or sprouting bag

1 ¼ - 1 ½ cups of sugar (400 grams or so)

¾ Gallon of filtered water

(more info on water, tea, and sugar follow this recipe)

A gallon jar (I get mine from bars; just ask the bartender or barback for an empty olive jar. A busy bar will throw away or recycle a few of these a week, so if you time it right they'll be happy to share. And if you're slowly sipping a dirty martini with extra olives and tip well, you might increase your chances)

Something to keep out bugs but let in air, like a sprouting bag, coffee filter or piece of clean cloth and rubber band

A bottle of kombucha (unpasteurized, unflavored)

What you'll do:

Clean your gallon jar with soap and hot water. You can sterilize it with UV light, H202, or an oven if you're nerdy by nature like me (see pg 75).

Heat about half of the water to almost boiling; remove from heat and stir in tea. If you heat 2 quart jars full of water in a microwave for 10 minutes then pour it into the gallon jug and brew right there, there's one less thing to wash. The hot, empty jars will quickly dry and be sparklingly clean.

After the tea has brewed sufficiently (some people go 5 minutes, others overnight) pour in the sugar and stir to dissolve it. Don't add the sugar to the boiling water because it will caramelize, though semi-hot water will help the sugar dissolve. Next add the rest of the water and let it cool to room temperature; there should be enough room at the top to allow for the kombucha starter and bubbles. Stick a clean finger in the tea to make sure it's comfortable to touch. If it's too hot for your skin, it's too hot for your new microscopic pets.

Pour in the bottle of kombucha tea, cover it with a coffee filter, clean cloth, or sprouting bag and let it sit in a warm place (60° F minimum, 75-80° F is optimal) for about 1 ½ - 2 weeks. Take a peek every so often and witness the awe-inducing formation of the SCOBY. If you haven't taken any creative license with these very lenient directions, you should have the beginnings of your own light-colored rubbery circle in a few days, and it should be fully formed in 1 ½ weeks or so. It looks like mold or curd as it's forming, don't fear, just wait and see that it forms a nice smooth disk. Taste the ferment. If it's sugar-sweet, that means that your little friends haven't eaten all the sugar and have some more work to do. The yeasts will actually produce fructose, or fruit sugar, which will be pleasantly sweet in a different way. If left to ferment further, they'll convert the fructose into gluconic and acetic acids, the flavors that give vinegar its kick. I like a good balance between the three, not too sweet with a nice acidic bite.

The brew is done when it's refreshingly sparkling, pleasant-tasting (as long as you like the taste of the tea you started with) and slightly acidic (a ph of around 3.5 for you sciencey types). Five minutes of work and a couple of weeks of waiting and you have a gallon of this probiotic and enzyme-rich elixir.

There are two different ways to continue your kombucha fun: when you get to the end of your gallon, save a little bit of the liquid, clean the jar, and start over from the beginning. The other way is to do a continuous ferment: adding the amount of tea that you remove every other day or so, an uninterrupted process. I prefer the second method for several reasons. There's no waiting involved – after you've taken out your tea for the day, add enough sweet tea to fill the jar back up and your already-existing SCOBY will immediately go to work on breaking it down, so it will be ready the next day. It's easier – very simple to make a few cups of tea and pour them into your jar, and there's no weekly cleaning necessary. It's more consistent - since you're just maintaining a powerfully established ferment, your brew is much less likely to be influenced by wild bacteria and yeasts. It's healthier – gluconic acid, the factor most responsible for kombucha's wonderful cleansing properties, doesn't appear until about a week and a half. Many other esoteric benefits don't develop until 2 or 3 weeks, or more.

When I was first fermenting kombucha, I used two 3-gallon glass jars with spigots that were sold as lemonade or vodka infusion jars on ebay. They were $18 each. I let one of them get about half empty, re-filled it with sweet tea, and then switched to drinking from the other one until it got half empty, going back and forth like this indefinitely. If you go out of town, bottle almost all the 'booch, cutting off the air and stopping the fermentation, and stick it in the fridge or take it with you. Use beer bottles with snap-on lids or old kombucha bottles with heavy-duty screw-on caps – both are made to withstand some pressure. You can also use wine bottles and pound the cork back in with a rubber mallet (synthetic corks work best). If you use a container with a metal cap, keep it stored upright so the acidic tea won't come in contact with it and eat away at the metal. When you're gone the tea still in the jars will become quite acidic, so when you get home and start 2 new batches of brew, it will be ready to drink quickly. This technique also works well if you have a surplus of finished brew. Stick your bottled tea in the fridge when it's at its peak, in your opinion, adding whole or pureed citrus, ginger, berries, herbs, or other flavorings for your personal peek at the sublime.

Secondary fermentation is what happens in the bottle with the cap on at room temperature. Without new oxygen, the yeasts become more active (as opposed to the bacteria, who were the star during open-air fermentation). The yeasts will continue to ferment any sugar left in your brew. Their waste product is carbon dioxide (the same thing that gives beer, champagne, and soda its bubbles), so as fermentation continues, the pressure will increase. Most people like to flavor their 'booch with 10-20% juice and leave their closed bottled out for a few days before sticking them in the fridge. Bottles can be "aged" for months or years, flavors developing and bubbles getting smaller and softer in the process, just like a fine champagne.

On Water, Tea, and Sugar

Water

Purified water is best for all the recipes in this book. Tap water contains many additives meant to kill off unwanted microorganisms in the water supply. These chemicals will also kill your kombucha culture, as well as the probiotics in your own system. Buying water or getting it delivered can be expensive, time-consuming, and environmentally unfriendly, and almost all bottled water is just filtered tap water in pretty bottles. If they're plastic bottles, they've been leaching chemicals into the water. The best route is to filter water yourself at home. A filtration system that removes chlorine, fluorine, chloramine, pesticide residue, heavy metals, and other contaminants can be had for a couple of hundred dollars; reverse osmosis is unnecessary unless you're using untreated water from a private well or spring. Distillation removes everything… For city-dwellers, carbon block or another simple filtration system that pulls water through a .5 – 1 micron screen is fine.

Though some municipalities use other sanitizers, chlorine is the most common and easy to get rid of. If tap water is your only option, pour a gallon into a pot and let it sit for a day; the chlorine, which is lighter than air, will evaporate out.

Tea

Black teas, such as Sencha or Darjeeling, are the standard for kombucha brewing, and they're what most commercial brewers use. They don't have to put this, or what kind of sugar they use, on the labels, as the kombucha is considered to convert them, which it does but not completely. Black tea is the fermented leaves of the tea plant, and has the highest caffeine content of any tea; about half of the caffeine in the original tea gets converted into the many acids listed above, and the other half remains in the brew. If you're sensitive to caffeine, green tea works just as well and has about a third the caffeine of black (as well as a host of anti-oxidant properties). Green tea is the unfermented, dried and steamed leaves of the tea plant. Black tea will produce a fruity, apple-y amber brew, while green will have a light and grassy flavor. Oolong tea is halfway between green tea and black tea, both in flavor and caffeine content. It's gently rolled after picking and allowed to partially ferment until the edges of the leaves start to turn brown.

Earl grey has bergamot oil which is damaging to the culture. Herbal teas will not work either, at least in the long run, because they have oils that could damage the culture, and are missing the nutrients and purines found in the tea plant that are necessary to produce the brew. There are two exceptions. Rooibos is a South African plant that is caffeine-free and is respected for its health benefits; it's anti-aging and anti-allergy, has oligosaccharides (compounds found to fight viral infections), combats high blood pressure, diabetes, and atherosclerosis, and is good for the skin. Honeybush is a different family of plants, though also from South Africa, and is slightly sweeter than rooibos. Neither rooibos nor honeybush contain tannins, so are fine for people with tannic allergies, and can be steeped much longer than true tea without becoming bitter.

Caffeine stimulates the reproduction of microorganisms, so if you're using a caffeine-free tea and find your fermentation slowing down, you may want to do a cycle of caffeine tea to re-invigorate your brew. It can be given away if you're sensitive or allergic to caffeine.

It's much cheaper to buy tea "loose", that is, not in bags, and measure the appropriate amount into a sprout bag or tea ball. A kitchen scale is invaluable for this, as well as measuring the sugar, herbs and spices, and mail (if you print your postage out from home on usps.com you get free tracking). They start at $15 with free shipping on ebay, and my cheap Chinese scale has lasted me 4 years thus far.

Sugar

White sugar, also called "evaporated cane juice" or other creatively green-washed derivatives, is the best for kombucha. It's sugar in its simplest form, which the simple digestive systems of single-celled organisms appreciate. Other sweeteners might be better for us, like honey, palm sugar, or molasses, but these are more difficult for the culture to utilize and leave residual substances in the brew, which can ferment on their own by attracting unwanted organisms. There will be some sugar leftover in the brew that you drink (though some of the sweetness comes from sugar recombined into the fruit sugar fructose), but it's a small price to pay for the innumerable benefits. Use organic, free-trade if possible, unbleached sugar (though not brown or muscovado).

Health Benefits of Kombucha

First off, kombucha is a living beverage, complete with all the enzymatic and probiotic benefits discussed elsewhere in this book. But that's not all – ferment now and we'll also throw in these powerful compounds...

LACTIC ACID is found in kombucha in its most potent form L-lactic(+). Lactic acid is essential for the digestive system in breaking down foods, improving digestibility, stimulating peristaltic movement of the intestines to improve regularity, assisting blood circulation, normalizing acidity of gastric juices, which in turn helps maintain proper body pH (see section on Alkalinity in "Kitchen Sink Farming Volume 1: Sprouting", pg 111), and helps restore the level of healthy bacteria in the digestive system. It's also highly detoxifying. Eli Metchnikoff won a Nobel Prize in 1908 for his research on the benefits of lactic acid to our health and immune system.

GLUCORONIC ACID is responsible for "xenobiotic metabolism" (from the Greek xeno, stranger) that remove toxic foreign substances from the liver like drugs, pollutants, androgens, estrogens, corticoids, and retinoids.

ACETIC ACID inhibits harmful bacteria in both you and your brew. It also gives the tea a nice kick. This is where the vinegar flavor comes from that will increase as the brew is fermented further.

MALIC ACID also assists in detoxification.

OXALIC ACID encourages the mitochondria, the cell's energy producer, and is a natural preservative.

GLUCONIC ACID is effective against many yeast infections such as candidiasis and thrush, and dissolves mineral deposits, those crunchy things that develop in chronically tight muscles.

BUTYRIC ACID is produced by the yeasts and when working with gluconic acid, also helps combat yeast infections such as candida.

NUCLEIC ACIDS work with the body in aiding healthy cell regeneration.

AMINO ACIDS are the building blocks of protein.

GLUCOSAMINES prevent or treat all forms of arthritis by increasing synovial hyaluronic acid production. This joint lubricant functions physiologically to aid in the preservation of cartilage structure and helps the joints glide, preventing arthritic pain. Hyaluronic acid and synovial fluid are the major difference between young joints and old ones, as this emollient decreases as we age. It enables connective tissue to bind moisture thousands of times its weight and maintain tissue structure, moisture, lubrication and flexibility, and elsewhere in the body lessens free radical damage while associated collagen retards and reduces wrinkles.

PROBIOTICS improve digestion, fight candida and other harmful yeasts, and remove carcinogens in the intestines and colon, fighting cancer in yet another way. These biologically active aspects of kombucha are being studied for their far-reaching effects, relieving everything from symptoms of fibromyalgia to depression and anxiety.

It's extraordinarily ANTIOXIDANT RICH, boosting the immune system in both the short and long terms, and increasing energy levels.

An in-depth study of several individual ferments found analgesic compounds, anti-arthritics, anti-spasmodics, hematinics (increase hemoglobin content of the blood so used to treat anemia, iron deficiency) and counteractions for hepatotoxins, anti-fungal compounds, and several anti-microbial/anti-bacterial compounds. They also contained beneficial enzyme inhibitors of glucuronidase, heparinase, hyaluronidase, and monoamine oxidase. But because kombucha is a living product resulting from the actions of dozens of organisms, what is in a ferment is not 100% universal, except for gluconic, acetic and glucuronic acids, and fructose.

Kombucha hasn't yet been extensively studied by medical science because of its relatively recent debut on the Western stage. But based on the Russian discovery that entire regions of their vast country were seemingly immune to cancer, researchers at the Hokkaido University in Japan have isolated either glucuronic or glucaric acids, substances which help the liver in detoxification. Without the presence of these compounds, the liver will re-absorb whatever toxin it has just laboriously removed from the blood and bowels. It's also rich in many of the enzymes and bacterial acids our bodies use for detoxification, thereby easing the workload on the liver, pancreas, blood, and digestive system. This family of substances is being looked into for its anti-cancer properties and seeming ability to render some chemotherapy-related toxins completely inert. There is, however, overwhelming anecdotal evidence about kombucha's anti-cancer properties. Alexander Solzhenitsyn, the recently deceased Russian author and Nobel prize winner, claimed in his autobiography that kombucha tea cured his stomach cancer during his internment in Soviet labor camps. Because of this testimony, President Ronald Reagan used kombucha to halt the spread of his cancer in 1987. He didn't die until 2004, and that was from age-related disease, not cancer.

Billions of microorganisms of different species working together to feed, nourish, cleanse, and sustain. I'll drink to that.

Kombucha can also be used to ferment other things in the same way that vegetables are "pickled" with raw apple cider vinegar. Fill a jar with sliced cucumbers and kombucha with onions, garlic, dill, and a grape leaf (for crunchiness) and enjoy fresh zingy pickles in a few days to a few weeks. Put a SCOBY and some starter tea in coffee for "Coffee-Boocha®", one of my probiotic drink company's most popular products (SOMA evolutionary refreshment in Portland, Oregon).

Jun

Very little is known about this very special culture, said to be from Tibet. It's hard to find, my company is the only one I know of producing it commercially, and I've never found any studies about it. Hard-core kombucha fans often try jun once and switch their allegiance, as jun gives a calm and grounded energy that's at the same time mellow and ecstatic.

While kombucha is a symbiotic colony of 30-40 different bacteria and yeasts, jun is just one of each. Jun lives on honey and green tea as opposed to kombucha's sugar and black tea craving, and their difference is evidenced by their nearly identical fermentation time – but brew kombucha with honey and you'll likely triple or quadruple your wait. Honey has powerful anti-bacterial properties, some of which are enzymatic and therefore destroyed by heating, but even cooked honey has a compound that's antibacterial. More on honey in the "Desserts" section of "Kitchen Sink Farming Volume 4: Living Homegrown Recipes – What to Do with Your Sprouts and Krauts".

Jun loves raw honey and takes on an appley-pear flavor as it brings out honey's malic and citric acids with a fructose boost - the combination that gives pears and apples their distinctive crisp sweetness - a process that also takes place in nice wines, though jun does it without making alcohol. It's interesting to note that kombucha doesn't like raw honey, and using it instead of sugar will slow kombucha's fermentation time to a month or longer (or kill the culture). Many jun cultures are actually kombucha, and fermenting speed is one way to test this. Jun SCOBYs also look darker, thinner, and less rubbery than kombucha's.

If you're lucky enough to find a jun mother, ferment it in the following manner:

Bring 3 liters of water to 200°F and remove from heat

Steep 12 Green Teabags (or 1 oz tea – twice as much as for kombucha) for 5-10 minutes

Add 2 Cups Honey (raw preferred, wait until water is under 110°F before adding)

When liquid is cooled to room temperature, add jun mother

Pour all into a gallon jar and cover with a clean cloth

Drink after a week or two, depending on temperature and strength of your culture. Jun is very sensitive and goes dormant or dead much more easily than any other culture, and may require some coaxing or another starter. When you have a strong culture going, put a mother in the freezer as a backup.

Kefir (Dairy)

Kefir is another "imported" culture; here it refers to dairy kefir. There's a culture called "tibicos" that ferments juice anaerobically (as opposed to dairy kefir, which uses oxygen) and is also referred to as "juice kefir" – more on this in the next section. Dairy kefir is a group of specific bacteria and yeasts that the inhabitants of the Caucus Mountains in Russia have asserted for centuries or more are responsible for their longevity. Like kombucha, the organisms responsible for making kefir form a polysaccharide mass, in this case fluffy cloud-like chunks that can grow to the size of garbanzo beans, called *kefir grains*, which give the probiotics something to attach to. The various cooperating microorganisms that make kefir occur naturally in the Caucuses; the story goes that the inhabitants of the region used to hang large leather sacs filled with milk in their doorways, organically inviting in the benevolent microscopic visitors; guests would give the bag a friendly slap or sharp poke on their way in and out and thereby keep the brew mixed and fermentation even. Those of us with Russian grandparents aren't surprised at the harshness sometimes shown to objects of love and affection.

Kefir has been much more thoroughly studied by medical science than kombucha (maybe because its effects were more localized and therefore more obvious), and the amount of hard data is encouraging. Dr. Orla-Jenson, a noted Danish bacteriologist specializing in dairy research states, "Kefir digests yeast cells and has a beneficial effect on the intestinal flora". It's high in calcium, amino acids, B-vitamins and folic acid, can repair a damaged digestive system or help build a healthy one in babies, and has even been shown to protect against the negative effects of nuclear radiation. If it can combat radiation imagine how powerful it can be against the effects of environmental damage, pollution, stress, harmful bacteria, viruses, fungi, and yeasts such as Candida, a harmful parasite that grows in the bloodstream of over 80% of people. Kefir's friendly cultures also produce specific antibiotic substances which can control undesirable microorganisms and act as anti-carcinogens. It's also been proven to combat acne in more than three-quarters of teenaged sufferers tested.

For people who drink milk, the benefits of kefir are mainly due to the breakdown of the aspects of milk that make it difficult to digest, thereby allowing all the benefits to be fully enjoyed. Lactose is converted into the immensely beneficial lactic acid, so people with lactose intolerance (an estimated 75% of the world's population) can enjoy kefir without digestive anxiety. It also pre-digests the many proteins, which no longer stay hard and are largely unusable by humans.

Eli Metchnikoff, an international Nobel Prize-winning researcher, found in 1908 that kefir activates the flow of saliva, most likely due to its lactic acid content and its slight amount of carbonation, and that it stimulates peristalsis (the wave-like motion of the bowels that push food along) and digestive juices in the intestinal tract. For these reasons, it is recommended as a post-operative food since most abdominal operations cause peristalsis (the waving motion of the bowels that pushes food through) to freak out and stop. It's also great to use whenever digestion has slowed, due to travel, stress, sleep deprivation, or pregnancy.

Dr. Johannes Kuhl conducted one of the foremost European studies of lactic acid, which he found in high amounts in kefir. Among many other benefits, he found that a well-balanced diet with liberal amounts of lactic acid fermented foods was a good protection against cancer.

For folks concerned about the safety of drinking milk that's been sitting out for days or weeks, it should be noted that lactic acid bacteria actually fight pathogenic organisms, killing e. coli and salmonella, while s. paratyphi and c. diphtheriae lose their pathogenic properties. Kefir cultures have also been reported to help treat achylia gastrica, peptic ulcers, cholecystitis, gastroenteritis, colitis, diarrhea, and dysentery.

Dairy Kefir: History and Mystery

The origins of kefir are shrouded in mystery and adventure. It was said to be given to the people of the northern slopes of the Caucasian Mountains by Mohammed, who told them to closely guard their secret, as the strength of this powerful health tonic would dissipate as more people learned about it. "The Grains of the Prophet" were seen as part of a family's wealth and were passed on from generation to generation like an heirloom, so for centuries the people of the northern Caucasus enjoyed this fizzy tonic and its benefits in secret.

Tales began to spread about kefir's existence, and Marco Polo mentioned a "magical" elixir of fermented milk in his writings. Most of the world remained largely ignorant of kefir, however, until the end of the 19th Century, when Russian doctors began studying the health of the people from the Caucus Mountains and deciding that kefir was worth looking into. Not being able to find a source for the grains, however, the All Russian Physician's Society enlisted the help of the Blandov Brothers, who not only ran the Moscow Dairy, but also had ties to the Caucus region. With the agreement that they would be the only commercial producers, the brothers became determined to procure some of the probiotic beverage.

In the summer of 1908 they sent a beautiful young employee, Irina Sakharova, to the court of a local prince, Bek-Mirza Barchorov. Her mission: charm the prince into giving away some kefir grains, and whisk them back to Moscow. The jealousy with which this mystical culture was guarded was underestimated, however, and when the prince discovered her plan he imprisoned her with a mind to keep her there, forever as his bride. A daring rescue by agents of the Blandovs followed, the forced marriage was stopped and the foiled prince dragged before the Czar. It was decided that Irina Sakharova was to be given ten pounds of the grains as recompense for her insults, and the Blandovs began the cultivation and production of kefir which is immensely popular in Moscow to this day.

In the 1970's and early 80's, microbiologists attempted to create kefir grains from the isolated organisms that make up the colony. They were unsuccessful, and it's still unknown how the bio-matrix that is a kefir grain is created. The researchers eventually gave up, capitulating to the fact that an unknown factor made the first propagation of kefir possible in the Caucus Mountains, for reasons that are unable to be duplicated in the lab.

Just as it was for the All Russian Physician's Society in the early 1900's, the hardest part for modern kefir cultures is finding the grains, but a quick internet search will yield lots of people willing to sell or share (check out the "Resources" section at the end of the book). Try to find grains that have been used in raw milk, which will be the strongest and most viable, with goat's milk preferred over cow's. I've never seen any that weren't grown in organic milk, but make sure to double check that. Gently put your grains in a glass jar, pour in some milk (again organic raw goat milk is best, but your kefir will improve any kind of milk), and cover the jar in a way that lets in air and keeps out bugs; the old sprout bag or coffee filter and rubber band or screw-on ring method works fine. The grains can also be used to make kefir out of nut and seed milks, coconut water or milk, fruit and vegetable juice, or even water with sugar, maple syrup, honey or other sweetener. I heard about some people who kefir-ed Gatorade, dyeing their grains a neon blue. This didn't change the culture's effectiveness but I wouldn't recommend that for obvious reasons. Kefir cultures thrive in mammal milk, however, and I recommend a cycle in raw animal milk for every couple of weeks in other liquids, though I've had a stable group of grains fermenting in coconut water for several months.

To make kefir, put a couple of tablespoons into milk (raw is best, and though it will ferment any mammal milk, goat is recommended over cow because of many reasons, such as its easier digestibility and better nutrition. For humans.). Cover the container with a clean cloth, sprout or produce bag, or coffee filter and secure it. Kefir stays un-refrigerated while it's brewing, and in a few hours to a day the whey will separate from the milk proteins, which rise to the top of the liquid, and a quick swirl or stir with a spoon or chopstick will blend them back together. I employ a continuous fermentation method like the one with kombucha.

Your kefir will be ready in a day or two – taste and smell your milk to determine readiness. When to enjoy your kefir is a matter of taste; the healthful lactic acid will produce a kind of sourness, so the kefir is done when it's the sourest you can enjoy. Then, just like with kombucha, you have the choice to do an interrupted or continuous fermentation – cover and put the finished kefir in the fridge and start a new batch, or every time you strain some kefir out, pour some fresh milk back in. About a half day later, the whey will separate out of the fresh milk; a swirl or stir will mix it back in. Just like with kombucha, I recommend the continuous process; it's easier, gentler on the culture, and I have to imagine that (again, just like kombucha) new benefits are continually created over the weeks and months. I've been using this method for years and my potent culture is consistent and dependable.

When you're ready to enjoy your kefir, strain some through a screen strainer into a glass, and gently drop the grains back into the fermenting culture. Or get a tea straw, like ones made for yerba mate or loose-leaf tea that has a little strainer at the bottom (glass is easy to keep clean), and just drink straight from your culture. Never rinse the grains or press them to squeeze out the kefir, as you're washing away valuable probiotics. The grains will increase in size and quantity; soon you'll notice your fermentations speeding up, and you'll have enough grains to separate for other fermenting projects, give away, or eat, as they happen to taste sweet and delicious. The kefir produces carbon dioxide, and putting an airtight lid on the finished product in the fridge will produce an effervescent potation.

I went through a phase of tossing kefir into most anything liquid I made: salad dressings, smoothies, dips and soups, slightly souring and adding a new dimension of flavor and health to each (check out the recipe for "Pepita Sour Crema" in "Kitchen Sink Farming Volume 4: Homegrown Living Recipes – What to Do with Your Sprouts and Krauts"). The kefir grains want to be able to get at all of the liquid; if it's so thick that there's no circulation, you'll just have a pocket of healthy fermentation happening in what's otherwise a jar of stuff sitting out on the counter. You want to avoid that so other bacteria don't come in and colonize the rest while the forces of good are trapped elsewhere. If the substance doesn't move freely, you'll want to stir it a few times a day with a spoon or chopstick, and in a few days it'll taste like you added goat cheese, sour cream, or yogurt to whatever you were using. The health benefits of this are obvious, but the culinary aspects can be quite pleasantly surprising: kefir'ed cream of mushroom soup and tomato-basil bisque (just to mention a couple) are so good you'll never want to go back to the ordinary versions. If you can't find the grains to remove them, don't worry about it; they're delicious and also very healthy.

Kefir grains are acidic, and for this reason many people recommend not using metal utensils thinking that the kefir will leach metals from the substance. This is true only in the case of reactive metals such as brass, aluminum, copper, silver, zinc, and iron. Stainless steel is fine. When kefir was catching on in the early 20th century, these reactive metals were commonly used to make kitchen implements, so that's maybe where the thought came from. I only say this as a warning not to bring the above metals in contact with your culture, and also in case someone tells you that all metal is a no-no, a common misconception.

Kefir Recap:

Add kefir grains to milk (1 tablespoon to a quart minimum, there's no maximum. More grains = faster fermentation)

When separation occurs, swirl or stir the brew to keep curds (floating proteins) and whey (clear liquid) together. In 1-3 days, strain out some kefir with a mesh strainer and dump the grains back in, or drink straight out of the jar with a straining straw, and refill with fresh milk

---

Kefir Part II

Your living ferment is a delicious and probiotic beverage on its own, but it's also a versatile starter culture for anything from apple butter to sauerkraut.

Living kefir separates into two parts: whey and laban. Whey, the clearish liquid that rises to the top of fermenting kefir, can be poured off and added to pretty much anything: chopped vegetables, like cabbage for kefir-kraut, and fruit butters are among my favorites - look for "Ginger-Kefir Apple Butter" in "Kitchen Sink Farming Volume 4: Homegrown Living Recipes – What to Do with Your Sprouts and Krauts".   Sulfur-containing amino acid-rich kefir whey can also be used in place of buttermilk in any recipe, or subbed for water in bread for an easy sourdough or even cake (see "Whey-Dough Bread" and "Sour Chocolate Cake" in "Kitchen Sink Farming Volume 4 – Homegrown Living Recipes – What to Do with Your Sprouts and Krauts). Whey-Good Ginger Cream Soda (pg 123) is much easier than capturing your own wild "ginger bug" and, as the name implies, the whey gives a delicious creaminess to the soda. Whey can also be used as a facewash, anti-dandruff shampoo, or mixed with aloe vera gel to make an emollient, anti-psoriasis lotion or shave cream. It can also be added to any drink or food for humans or animals for a nutritive probiotic boost.

Whey can be added to cream to make sour cream, which can then be shaken or churned to make real olde-timey butter (next section).

What's left after the whey and grains are removed is called "laban", or Basic Kefir Cheese, and is the other starter in kefir. The best way to remove all the whey is to pour the strained kefir into a sprout bag or pre-moistened cheesecloth, and hang it over a bowl for 12-24 hours. It can also be done in smaller quantities in a coffee-maker – spoon some kefir onto a coffee filter and put the coffee pot underneath to catch the whey.

The resulting laban is a flavorful cross between cream and cottage cheese, and is awesome right away, spread on sprouted loaves, with fruit (a traditional dessert from the Caucuses), or any other way you'd use the previously mentioned condiments. Blend 3 tablespoons oil per cup of Basic Kefir Cheese, along with herbs or vegetables for a delicious dip. Plain Basic Kefir Cheese can also be used to make hard cheeses.

Add a teaspoon of salt to each quart of Basic Kefir Cheese, and put it back in the sprout bag, cheesecloth, or coffee filter. Osmosis will pull even more liquid out, and another day of draining will yield a nice block of cheese that can be pressed into a wheel or brick and left to air dry for a week7 or two. To give it just a little air, put it into a sprout bag in a jar, hang the string over the lip of the jar, and screw the lid on. It can also be left on a counter with an upturned container over it, flipped daily. If a white mold covers the cheese, consider yourself lucky, as you have not one but two kingdoms of organisms working for your dinner: bacteria and mold. The white fuzz is harmless and will add a magnificent depth of flavor to your fromage. If the mold starts to get colorful though, these could be pathogens (probably not, but it's hard to test outside of a lab) so it's best to toss it and start over.

When the Basic Kefir Cheese is dry to the touch, it can be waxed to ripen without drying further (in two months you'll have a sharp cheddar, in 6 months to a year you'll get a robust parmesan). For kefir feta, drop your fresh cheese in a 7% salt-water solution for two months (make sure it's dry and well-pressed prior to plunking it in the brine so it doesn't fall apart). A little blue cheese can be mixed into the Basic Kefir Cheese and it will propagate into the whole thing. Most hard cheeses are best after at least two months of aging.

Storing your kefir grains

If you'll be away for a week or less, your kefir grains will hibernate nicely sealed in the fridge in some fresh milk. The fermentation will slow greatly, so to them it'll feel like a day on the counter. If you're leaving for 2 months or less, the grains can be frozen in a sealed container – a little dry milk powder will help prevent freezer burn. Frozen kefir has been known to last a year or more, but the best way to suspend your culture for the long-term is to dehydrate the grains. They can be dried at under 110° F for a couple of days until they look like little yellow lava rocks.

I find that drying them in a batch of kefir laban, spread out on a dehydrator sheet, helps them re-animate the fastest and most consistently.

Whey-Good Ginger Cream Soda

Ingredients:

1 ½ cups kefir whey
1 cup water
2 inches juiced or blended and strained ginger
4 Tbl sweetener – raw honey, sugar, etc.
1/2 tsp salt

Do:

Combine all ingredients in a quart or larger mason jar. Cover with a clean cloth, sprout or produce bag, or coffee filter, and allow to ferment at room temperature for 2-3 days. Optional: add juice of 5 oranges for a creamsicle treat.

Tibicos (Juice Kefir)

There exists another culture called water kefir or tibicos, and is from Japan. Like dairy kefir and kombucha, it makes a SCOBY, a symbiotic collection of bacteria and yeast, held together by a polysaccharide matrix. Water kefir SCOBY looks more like small clear crystals than rubbery rice-like dairy kefir grains, so for the sake of clarity I call it water kefir, crystal kefir, or tibicos, while dairy kefir retains the generic label "kefir".

Water kefir can live in any sugary liquid, producing readily available lactic acid bacteria and carbonation, and are the best choice for fermenting non-dairy beverages. These drinks will have less health benefits than kombucha and milk kefir, but coconut water "champagne" and fermented juices and teas are a wonderful way to enjoy cultured thirst-quenchers. Water kefir is also a great way to remove sugars from sweet liquids. I always crystal kefir maple syrup for the master cleanse (a ten-day diet of maple syrup, lemon juice, and cayenne in water to purify the digestive system and detoxify the body). My probiotic drink company, SOMA Evolutionary Refreshment® makes "Maharaj Cleanse®", a crystal kefired and kombuchaed master cleanse with the addition of crystal kefired coconut water, and it's very popular as both a cleanse and a beverage.

To make a sparklingly alive water kefir drink, gently drop a tablespoon or more of the grains into a juice, tea, or other liquid. Unless your liquid is naturally sweet, add a little sugar, raw honey, maple syrup or other sweetener, and seal. In 12-24 hours, the juice or sweetened tea will be slightly effervescent and alive. Strain the crystals out with a strainer. Your finished crystal kefir can be put in the fridge to slow the fermentation.

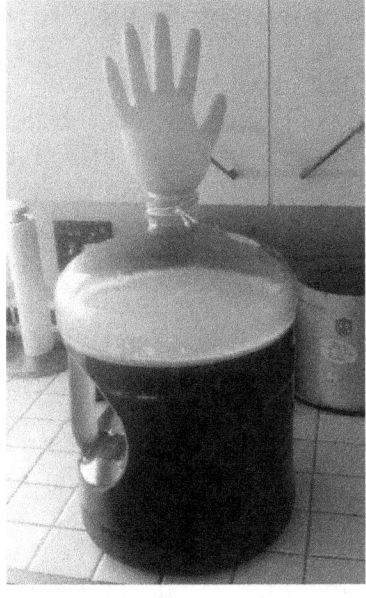

Kefiring maple syrup with an airlock from a surgical glove

The above process will

slowly make more kefir crystals as time goes by; if you'd like to make a lot fast there's another process: put your kefir crystals in a quart jar, add a cup of maple syrup, fill with filtered water and screw the lid on. This can be left indefinitely (open the top periodically to release pressure) and the grains will quickly multiply, making a thick crystally mud which will grow into crystals by the day.

Crystal kefiring maple syrup, 1 part syrup (organic grade B) to 2 or 3 parts filtered water or coconut water. This polycarbonate container can't take much pressure so will explode after a certain point. To keep the fermentation anaerobic, use an airlock or a balloon. I like to use a surgical glove so I'll be greeted by various gestures as the pressure increases. I've since found a source for glass 5-gallon containers and switched to using those.

Fermenting Fats – Butter and Oil

Butter has been enjoyed for as long as milk-producing animals have been domesticated – it's a natural by-product of raw milk and an effective way to store milk fat without refrigeration. If you let un-homogenized milk (milk that hasn't been crushed, turning the components into an undifferentiated liquid of deteriorating nutrition) sit out for a few hours you'll notice the fat globules, which are lighter than the protein and water that constitute the rest of the milk, rise to the top.

In our kefir-making, we stir or swirl to keep all parts together, but the milk fat can also be skimmed off of the surface, becoming cream. This is just what prehistoric man did, right before they beat it with sticks (how they started doing this I'll never know), until the fat globules stuck together and the protein-rich liquid, the buttermilk, was released. Their cream was already fermented by the wild lactic-acid bacteria in the environment, and in fact *all* butter was fermented for flavor and stability until the 1940's and the advent of butter-making machines. While cream needs a day or so to ferment and release its wonderfully rich flavor, the machines weren't going to run only half the time. Unfermented "sweet cream" butter was continuously "churned out" (sorry), and people got used to the flavor, soon forgetting the ancient heirloom goodness of traditional butter.

In the 1915 *Principles and Practices of Butter Making* by McKay and Larson, there's no mention of sweet cream butter.

"To Produce Flavor and Aroma: The chief object of cream-ripening is to secure the desirable and delicate flavor and aroma which are so characteristic of good butter. These flavoring substances, so far as known, can only be produced by a process of fermentation. It is a well-known fact that the best flavor in butter is obtained when the cream assumes a clean, pure, acid taste during the ripening. For this reason, it is essential to have the acid-producing germs predominate during the cream ripening; all other germs should, if possible, be excluded or suppressed. When cream has been properly ripened, it is practically a pure culture of lactic-acid-producing germs, while sweet unpasteurized cream contains a bacterial flora, consisting of a great many types of desirable and undesirable germs."

Good news: your kefir culture is the perfect starter for making fermented butter, a fun and delicious process.

Making Butter:

Obtain raw cream, the higher the fat content the better the butter, and even though goat's milk is more nutritious than cow's, easier to digest and lighter in flavor, it's actually slightly higher in fat as well.

Put a few tablespoons of kefir whey into each cup of cream and stir well. Leave it to ferment for a day or two, or longer. I've gone up to two weeks (on a roadtrip) and the butter was amazing. Stir a few times a day - the cream is thick and the kefir has a harder time swimming around. You want every corner of the cream to be fermented.

Next, spoon the fermented cream into a jar or bottle with a tight fitting lid. It may seem counterintuitive in the next step, but the fuller the container, the faster the butter will come.

Now – shake shake shake. Just like our thick-browed ancestors did with their sticks, we're smacking the fat globules together, smashing their protein sheaths apart and letting the pieces get carried away in the water. In about ten or twenty minutes of hard shaking you'll have whipped cream, which (sorry) is even harder to shake. But keep at it - perseverance will soon yield small yellow lumps. Keep shaking and soon all of the milk fat will be separated from the buttermilk, which will look like floating yellow tapioca. Scoop it out, squish it into a ball and squeeze out the remaining liquid, and pat yourself on the back, if your arms can still move.

The paddle of a kitchen mixer can also do the job, as can a bunch of friends at a party or a kindergarten classroom passing the jar around. I've heard that butter was discovered by camel-riding traders in North Africa – when they reached their destination, they opened their pouches of raw milk and by the many steps of their beasts, butter happened. A jar of milk in the pocket of a long-distance hiker will meet a similar fate if their gait is bouncy enough.

Ghee

Native to the Himalayans, ghee is "clarified butter", or butter that's had the protein and water removed, leaving only the fat. Ghee contains all the nutritive benefits of butter and none of the casein and lactose, so it's easier to digest for many people. Because it's 100% fat, ghee will last a long time at room temperature, even unfermented. In Ayurvedic medicine, India's ancient "science of life", ghee is said to coat the nadis, the channels by which life force flows through the body, strengthening the energy field around the body, or aura. Because ghee is a simpler and therefore more easily digestible form of butter, its benefits to both the cardiovascular system and mental functioning are obvious to even more linear logic...

Traditionally, ghee is made by heating butter (made from yogurt) until the water evaporates out and the protein rises to the top and can be skimmed off. But we Kitchen Sink Farmers know better. Put butter in a dehydrator for a couple of days, and as the water vanishes, a white foam will form. Scoop it out as it grows (the liquid also can be strained at the very end to remove all traces of milk proteins) and you'll soon have unpasteurized, fermented, raw clarified butter. It's the best fat for cooking, if you do that, because ghee has one of the highest smoke points of all fats - 485° F. Scrumptious brushed on sprouted loaves or lightly dehydrated veggies, ghee's concentrated flavor from lack of water means that you need much less of it than butter in any food prep.

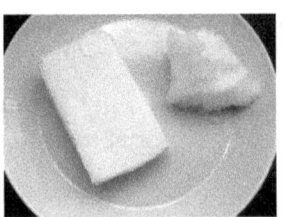

And Now The Crown Jewel of Fat... (and I don't mean Miss Piggy's Tiara)

The two healthiest fats together at last: kefir ghee and coconut oil. Coconut oil's succulent velvet added to ghee's nutty smoothness is, IMO, the quintessence of oils.

Coconut oil is the most processed food that comes into my kitchen. By this point, you know that I always start with whole foods, which I then attempt to use in a way that maximizes their nutrition, life force, and flavor. Coconut oil is something I don't often do at home[5], and I won't be without its many incredible health benefits and unbelievable flavor. Coconut oil fuses seamlessly into everything from dressings, smoothies, soups, and nut butters. It egolessly improves the flavor without trumpeting its presence.

Homemade butter and coconut oil

Coconut oil helps normalize blood lipids, protecting against damage to the liver by alcohol and other toxins, and in small amounts prevents kidney and gall bladder diseases. It's associated with the prevention and management of diabetes through its ability to stabilize blood sugar and regulate insulin production. Coconut oil has anti-viral, anti-

---

[5] Make coconut oil by dehydrating freshly shredded coconut meat (store-bought coconut flakes have been de-fatted). Blend the dried shreds in a high-speed blender and sit the paste ontop of a dehydrator or other warm place for a day or 2. The oil will rise to the surface, ready to be scooped off and enjoyed.

bacterial and anti-fungal properties, improves mineral absorption (which is important for all body processes including healthy teeth and bones), and is also the world's best skin and face lotion.

It's important to use organic coconut oil, as conventionally-produced products use all sorts of nasty chemicals and can be exposed to pathogens. Raw is even better, assuring the quickest and most gentle processing. My favorite brands are Nutiva, sold on amazon, and Hummingbird (www.hummingbirdwholesale.com), only available in stores. Nutiva has a raw, in glass, coconut oil but their basic oil is so well-prepared that I don't think the considerable extra expense is worth it. Look for the amazing price on two 54 oz. tubs. Hummingbird's raw, organic extra virgin oil is incredible, packed in glass instead of plastic, and among the cheapest coconut oils I've seen. If you can find it near you, do.

As a saturated fat, coconut oil is solid at room temperature[6], so in colder seasons I leave mine on top of my dehydrator or fridge so it's always liquid. Pour it into liquid ghee, in whatever ratio you like, stirring every so often as the mixture solidifies to keep them from separating.

---

[6] (<76°F, actually). Saturated fats have only single bonds in their carbon chains which allows them to be neatly "packed". Unsaturated fats have a double bond along their row of carbon, causing it to have a kink. Because of this bend, these molecules can't stack so easily and remain liquid at room temperature. Saturated fats, because of their ability to stack so easily, build up more quickly in the body than unsaturated fats. That's why in large quantities (especially with saturated fats derived from animals) this can be harmful to the body - these fatty acids can build up on the heart and blood vessels and affect their function.

Raw Fats and Unrefined Oils for Weight-Loss and Well-Being

Lipase, the enzyme that breaks down fats and is missing from refined oils and pasteurized dairy products, is vital for health. It's not only a major player in fat diseases like obesity, heart disease, diabetes, stroke, Parkinson's and degenerative muscle disease, but is also a factor in skin problems, autoimmune diseases, cancer, degenerative diseases of the brain and nervous system, and supports general rejuvenation and regeneration.

Fats and oils are not only essential for our energy metabolism, but they also play an important role in the structural integrity of our body. Most of our brain, nerves and cell membranes consist of fats, or "lipids". Lipase is important in maintaining optimal cell membrane permeability, allowing adequate nutrient supply into the cells and wastes to flow out. P.G. Seeger, the world's leading researcher on the relationship between nutrition and cancer has clearly shown that the first biochemical step towards cancer is a deterioration of the cell membrane.

As we age, the functioning of our pancreas, the body's lipase factory naturally declines. Decreasing lipase production leads to reduced bile flow and less surface area in the intestines for nutrient absorption. The resulting deficiencies of fat-soluble vitamins such as A, D, and E, phospholipids and essential omega-3-fatty acids in turn, contribute to the common symptoms of aging and the development of degenerative diseases, such as aging skin, Alzheimer's disease, arteriosclerosis and atherosclerosis, auto-immune disease, cancer, cardiovascular disease, chronic fatigue syndrome, cystic fibrosis, dementia, depression, diabetes, eye diseases, fibromyalgia, lateral sclerosis (A.L.S.), liver diseases, malabsorption of nutrients, multiple sclerosis, muscular dystrophy, obesity, pancreatitis, Parkinson's disease, psoriasis, Raynaud's disease, stroke, and vertigo.

Fat vs. Weight

With a strong metabolism, we can easily gain or lose weight. Two-thirds of US adults and one-third of children are now classified as overweight. Research shows that lipase deficiency is a huge factor in this alarming state of affairs.

The problem is this: the less fat there is in a meal, the more quickly it is released from the stomach into the small intestine. The plentiful carbohydrates that might be present in the same meal rush past the scanty and slow-moving fats and are rapidly absorbed into the bloodstream, which can lead to damaging high blood-sugar levels. In an effort to prevent this, the pancreas releases large amounts of insulin. This helps glucose enter cells more quickly but if you are not doing hard work or exercise at the time, the excess glucose is either converted to lactic acid (some of which is used by the brain, intestines, and red blood cells), thereby causing overacidity and mineral deficiency, or the glucose is converted to fat.

Fat is then stored in fat cells. When the blood sugar level drops, this stored fat can now be used to generate energy – but only if there is sufficient internal lipase. If lipase is deficient, fat remains in the fat cells and you need more readily-available energy, and so feel hungry again, having another carbohydrate meal with a replay of the same story. After several years of repeating this cycle with habitually elevated blood sugar levels, diabetes is often the result.

This finely-tuned system was designed under two assumptions: 1) humans lead an active lifestyle, especially when eating large amounts of starches, and 2) we eat unrefined, living fats - with lipase intact. These factors could be counted on in our ancestors' lives, but as the speed of changing culture has outrun the rate of genetic evolution, for the first time in our planet's history, a species has outsmarted it's own genetic mandate, with disastrous consequences.

Lipase-rich raw butter, for instance, is effective in the fights against psoriasis and tuberculosis, but (lipase-deficient) pasteurized butter can cause or aggravate them. The same is true for heart and liver problems, which are created or aggravated by processed cheese and butterfat. These health problems were less common in the centuries before pasteurization, and in the modern-day inhabitants of the Caucasus region with their high intake of raw milk products. Cholesterol was a non-issue in the old days when mainly unheated milk products were used, and cardiovascular disease was almost unknown. This was not because of lack of medical knowledge. Carnivorous wild animals have diets high in fat and cholesterol but show no signs of atherosclerosis and heart disease. In contrast, domesticated dogs and cats that live on canned food, pasteurized milk or cooked meat develop the same diseases as their caretakers.

There are two ways to solve this problem, and it's best to use both. First, get plenty of lipase, preferably from raw fats and oils, or there are also lipase supplements. Second, slow down the absorption of carbohydrates. There are 2 ways to do this: either eat less carbohydrates, or slowing down the emptying of the stomach by mixing carbohydrates with sufficient oil or fat. For example, eat fruit mixed with raw coconut or kefir, or grains mixed with raw oils or ghee.

Alternatively, one can eat mainly slow-digesting carbohydrates, such as sprouted legumes like garbanzos, mung beans or lentils, with vegetables and a raw oil-rich dressing. Another option that's very effective in bodies used to holding onto fat is snacking – small amounts of food at a time to space out the starch intake and absorption. Ingest only as much carbohydrate as you need to produce energy during the next 30 to 60 minutes so that nothing is converted into fat. Then have another snack. Finally, be aware that if you do have a high-calorie meal in the evening your body may have no choice but to store it in fat cells. Fat burning can also be accelerated by drinking enzyme- and probiotic-rich apple cider vinegar before meals.

All raw lipid-rich foods are high in lipase. However, lipase is water-soluble so it breaks down quickly without the protection offered by whole foods. There's not much lipase in pure oils; unless extremely fresh, the lipase in even unrefined oils breaks down quickly. This includes avocado oil and coconut oil.

In order to obtain a high lipase intake from vegetable sources, we need to consume the whole food. This means eating the avocado instead of using just the oil, or pressing, juicing or blending the coconut flesh to make and use coconut milk or cream. This needs to then be refrigerated or frozen because the high enzyme content causes it to deteriorate rapidly at room temperature.

This is not a problem with fresh olives, avocado, coconut flesh or raw dairy as they usually retain enough water and therefore, most of their lipase. Cream, for instance, has about 60% water, about 16% butter and about 50% egg yolk. Besides a diet high in refined and salty carbohydrates, the government ban on raw dairy products has done the most towards creating the epidemic of obesity in the country. The lawmakers can't be blamed, however, as they represent (usually) what their constituents want, or will accept. It started with the use of non-organic farming methods, leading to the breakdown of the immune systems in plants which were then not able to support a healthy immune system in dairy cows, and pathogens began to flourish. Chemical fertilizers and pesticides became commonplace because their use was accepted by the public and our "magic bullet" mentality, but long-term observation proves that quick-fixes rarely last.

Raw milk is illegal in many places, so dairy farmers that still understand the benefits of unadulterated milk have found creative solutions for getting real dairy to people. A popular method is "herd sharing", in which consumers will buy a "share" of a dairy animal, whether cow or goat, and have access to milk for a feed or packaging fee. Look at www.realmilk.com for herd shares in your area.

Oil-rich nuts and seeds are another great source of lipase, but need to be sprouted to receive the full benefit (see Kitchen Sink Farming Volume 1: Sprouting). Lipase is also available in supplement form, but is of course not as effective as a whole food source.

Fats and oils, or fatty foods such as egg yolk, ingested without thoroughly chewing together with other food (and thereby emulsifying it with the natural co-factor lecithin) are not absorbed efficiently and may cause indigestion and deficiencies. If, for example, you just swallow capsules of fish oil or vitamin E, or a spoonful of cod liver oil, the oil may just remain in a puddle and not be absorbed because lipase cannot penetrate. Always try to emulsify oils and fats by shaking them with lecithin, or the natural way, by thoroughly chewing them in their whole food forms.

Recommended Reading

Fermentation:

The Art of Fermentation: An In-Depth Exploration of Essential Concepts and Processes from Around the World by Sandor Ellix Katz and Michael Pollan

Wild Fermentation by Sandor Ellix Katz *with an incredible recommended reading list

Understanding: Bacteria Discovery Education School (DVD, and on youtube)

Sprouting:

Sprouts: The Miracle Food: The Complete Guide to Sprouting by Steve Meyerowitz and Michael Parman

The Sprouting Book: How to Grow and Use Sprouts to Maximize Your Health and Vitality by Ann Wigmore

The Wheatgrass Book: How to Grow and Use Wheatgrass to Maximize Your Health and Vitality by Ann Wigmore

Gardening:

Fresh Food from Small Spaces: The Square-Inch Gardener's Guide to Year-Round Growing, Fermenting, and Sprouting by R.J. Ruppenthal

Dirt: the Ecstatic Skin of the Earth by William Bryant Logan

Vegetarianism, Veganism, and Raw Food Prep:

Eating Animals by Jonathan Safran-Foer.

Diet for a New America and The Food Revolution by John Robbins.

Beyond Beef: The Rise and Fall of the Cattle Culture by Jeremy Rifkin

RAW by Charlie Trotter

Ani's Raw Food Kitchen: Easy, Delectable Living Foods Recipes by Ani Phyo

Environment, GMOs, and Agribusiness:

The Power of Community: How Cuba Survived Peak Oil (DVD and on youtube)

The Weather of the Future by Heidi Cullen

Stolen Harvest: The Hijacking of the Global Food Supply by Dr. Vandana Shiva

The World According to Monsanto (DVD)

Evolution and Pleasure

Stumbling on Happiness by Daniel Gilbert

How Pleasure Works by Paul Bloom

Supernormal Stimuli: How Primal Urges Overran Their Evolutionary Purpose by Deidre Barrett

Resources:

Seeds, Grains and Nuts:

NutsOnline.com - A family business with great prices, customer service, and a touch of whimsy in everything they do. They once sent a stuffed elephant with my order. Sold.

Wheatgrasskits.com - A great source for certain seeds as well as sprouting supplies.

Nutiva - The best hemp seeds and coconut oil. I get the 3-lb bag of organic shelled hempseeds and double pack of 54-oz jars of organic coconut oil, and I buy them through amazon.com to get free shipping and a "Subscribe and Save" discount. They also make a raw coconut oil which comes in glass and is great, and more expensive.

Sprouting Bags – available from great companies like Pure Joy Planet, but I use reusable mesh produce bags that are about 20 times cheaper and might last longer, but have a slightly wider mesh so the tiniest seeds like amaranth need the real deal. Or panty hose.

Probiotic Cultures

Dairy Kefir - kefirlady.com – a great source for dairy kefir grains grown in organic raw goat's milk, and at the time of this writing she sells a ¼ cup for $20 with shipping; top-quality grains at the best price on the net for the quantity. Is also very available to answer questions and share the enthusiasm.

Kombucha, Juice Kefir, Apple Cider Vinegar – try your local craigslist first, then ebay. Can also be started from a raw and unflavored product from your local natural foods store.

Index

Stay Connected!

Visit

www.KitchenSinkFarming.org

for tips, recipes, news, giveaways, and general delicious nerdiness.

www.ingramcontent.com/pod-product-compliance
Lightning Source LLC
Chambersburg PA
CBHW070653290526
45790CB00001B/294